Malcolm Finney
medical detective

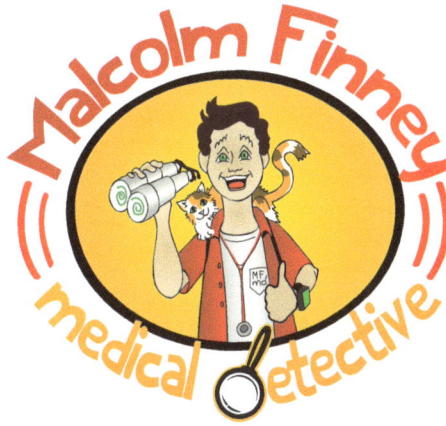

THE CASE of...
SUGAR MONSTER

Written By: **Erika Kimble**

Illustrated By: **Laurel Winters**

Bandages & Boo-Boos Press

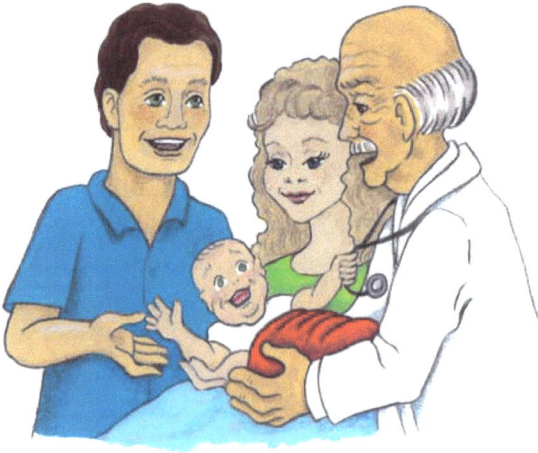

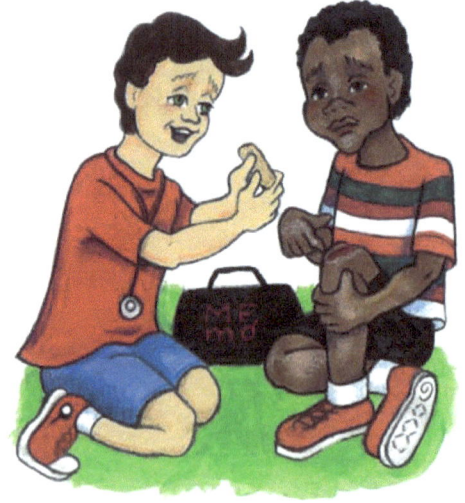

DEDICATION

To one of my best friends Nina, for being an inspiration to maintain a healthy lifestyle. As always, to my husband and babies, for inspiring me to live every day better. And to our nation's children: changing this epidemic begins with you! – E.K.

DEDICATION

To all "My Guys" for the joy they bring to my life. – L.A.W

ACKNOWLEDGEMENTS

Thank you to our content experts:
Dr. Ellen Rome, M.D., Dr. Karen Vargo, M.D.,
Amy Chand M.S., E.P., and Amy Headings, Ph.D., RD, LD.

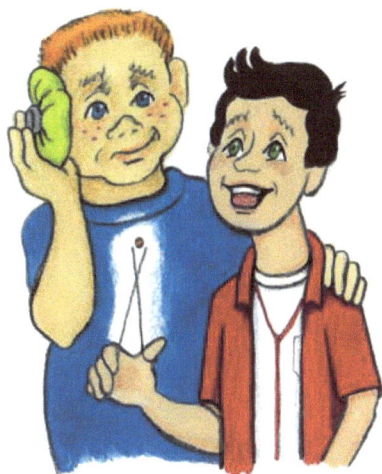

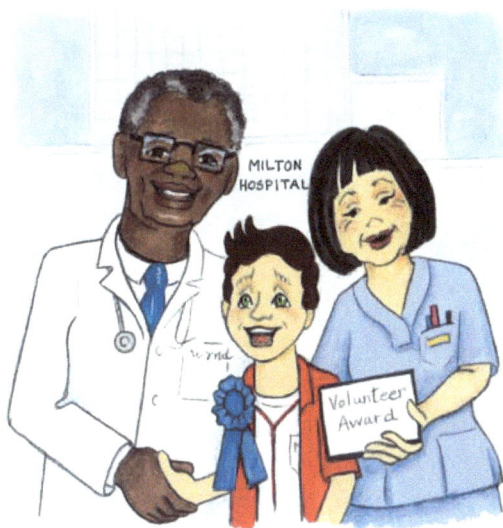

Book © 2013 Bandages & Boo-Boos Press
Text copyright © Erika Kimble 2013.
Illustrations copyright © 2013 by Laurel Winters.
Designed by: Jameson McMaster

All inquiries should be addressed to: **Bandages & Boo-Boos Press, LLC.**
9811 W. Charleston Blvd., Ste. 2-398,
Las Vegas, NV 89117
www.bandagesandbooboos.com

Printed in The United States of America.
Library of Congress Control Number: 2013918704
ISBN: 978-09859508-1-1

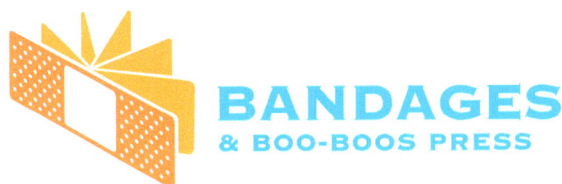

BANDAGES
& BOO-BOOS PRESS

AUTHOR'S NOTE

For Parents, Teachers, Caregivers, Librarians, Health Professionals, Families, Friends, and Others who Promote Health Education for Children.

Children are curious about their own bodies and differences they see in others. As a parent, I have experienced the embarrassing public moments of my son's stares and nudging, alerting me to a person with a medical condition. I then try to explain a complex illness in a way a young child can understand. Many parents or others who work with kids may find this scenario familiar. The Malcolm Finney book series was developed to address this curiosity. My hope is that children may become medical detectives, as they journey with Malcolm to understand diseases and variations in the human body. Malcolm Finney has been created for the child who can read and is beginning to ask and understand "Why?"

This series unfolds the answers to difficult questions with the belief that kids can be empowered to learn about differences and improve the health of themselves and others. Although this educational process is one that never ends, my hope is that the knowledge gained creates a foundation for a healthier, happier, future.

Sincerely,

Erika Kimble

Erika Kimble M.A., M.S., CNP

CONTENT

Malcolm cheered as the Milton Moose team swished a three-point goal just before the buzzer. The Milton Moosettes thundered across the arena and Malcolm waved to his best friend Carlita. Half-time vendors roamed the stairwells and an aroma of chocolate drifted by. The smell grew stronger as a boy carrying a snack tray trudged up the stairs.

"Looks like another medical mystery on the horizon," said Malcolm. "Not to worry: MALCOLM FINNEY, MEDICAL DETECTIVE, to the RESCUE!"

Get your freshly made cupcakes... (gasp), krispie treats... (gasp), brownies... (gasp). I can't make it up another flight of stairs.

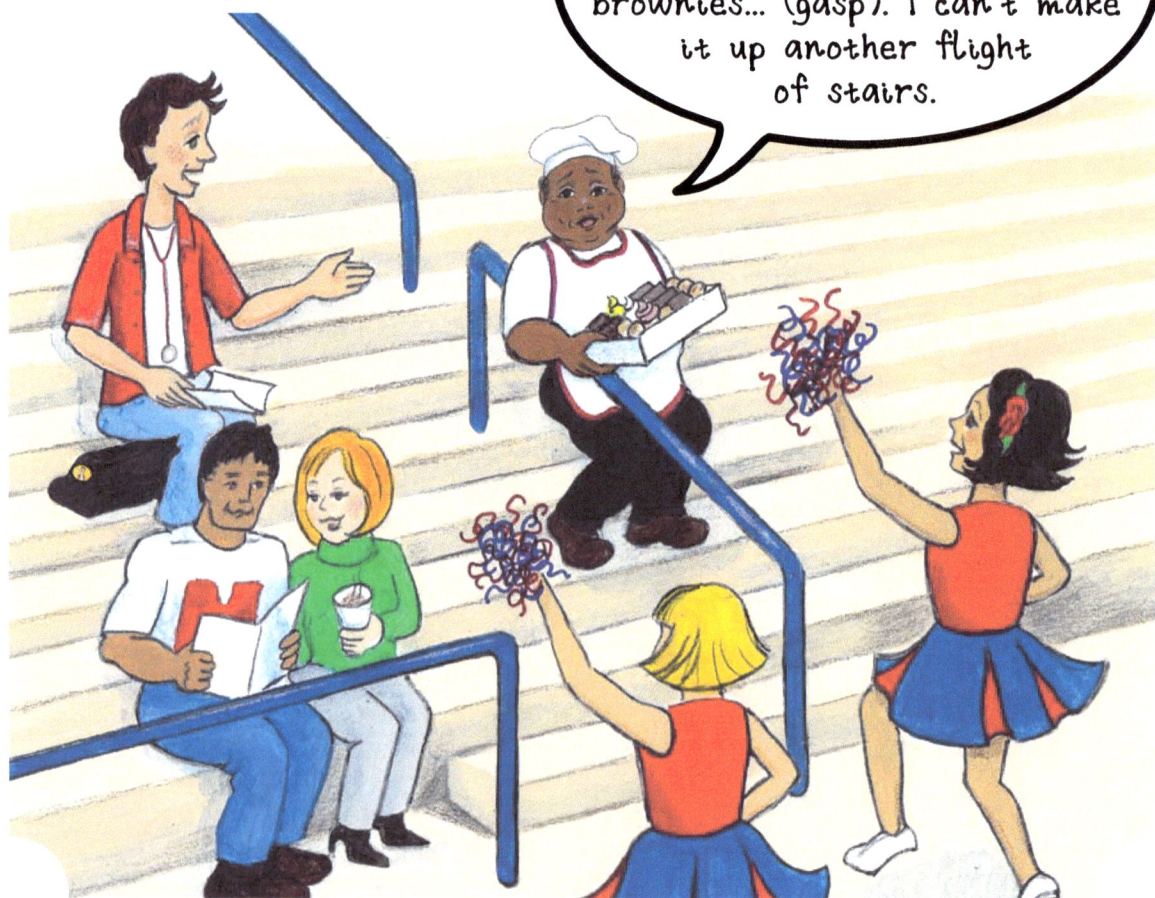

An ordinary fourth grader would have bought a cupcake, but Malcolm was no ordinary fourth grader. As a medical detective, he helped those in need whenever duty called - even during his friend's Moosette routine.

Let me help you.

Thanks. This tray gets heavy. I'm Lee, but people call me Sugar because I love to bake. I created Milton's famous Triple Chocolate Threat Brownie recipe.

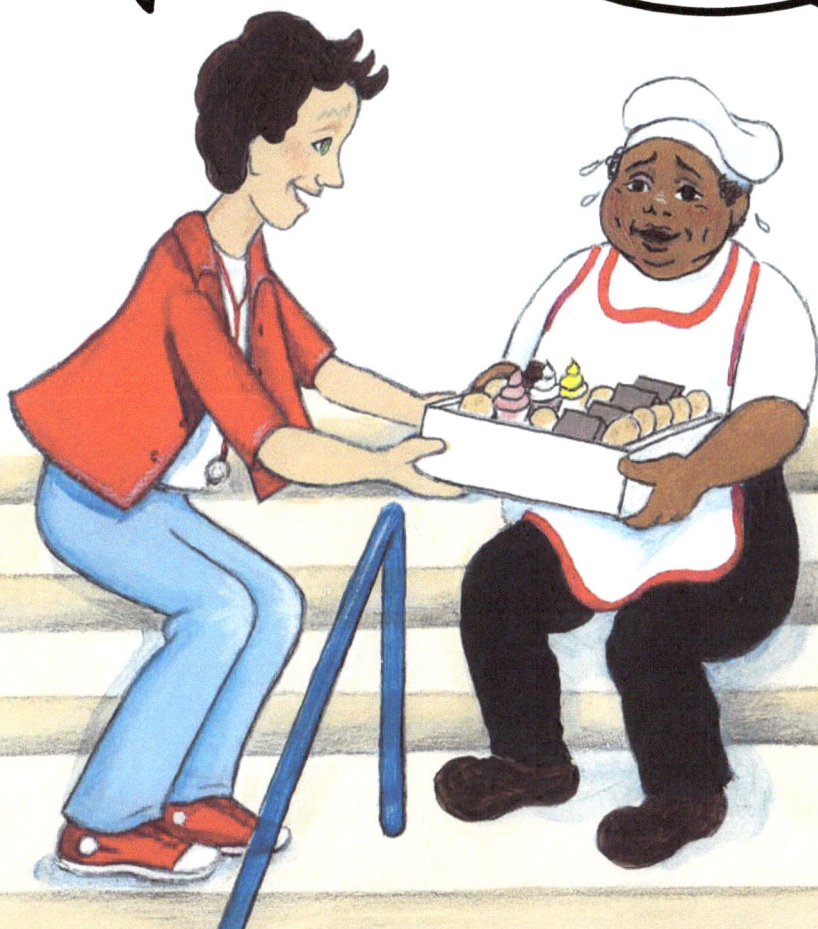

At the end of half-time, the crowds returned to their seats and Carlita ran up the stairs to assist Malcolm.

"I saw you struggling to carry your tray," said Carlita. "I thought you two could use a little assistance from your local inventor."

"Carlita," said Malcolm. "This is the gastronomical genius Sugar Lee, the creator of my favorite brownie! He has a mechanical dilemma that strains his back. Luckily, you're just the girl to fix it!"

"Any help would be great," said Sugar. "Especially with the big Ice Festival Competition coming up."

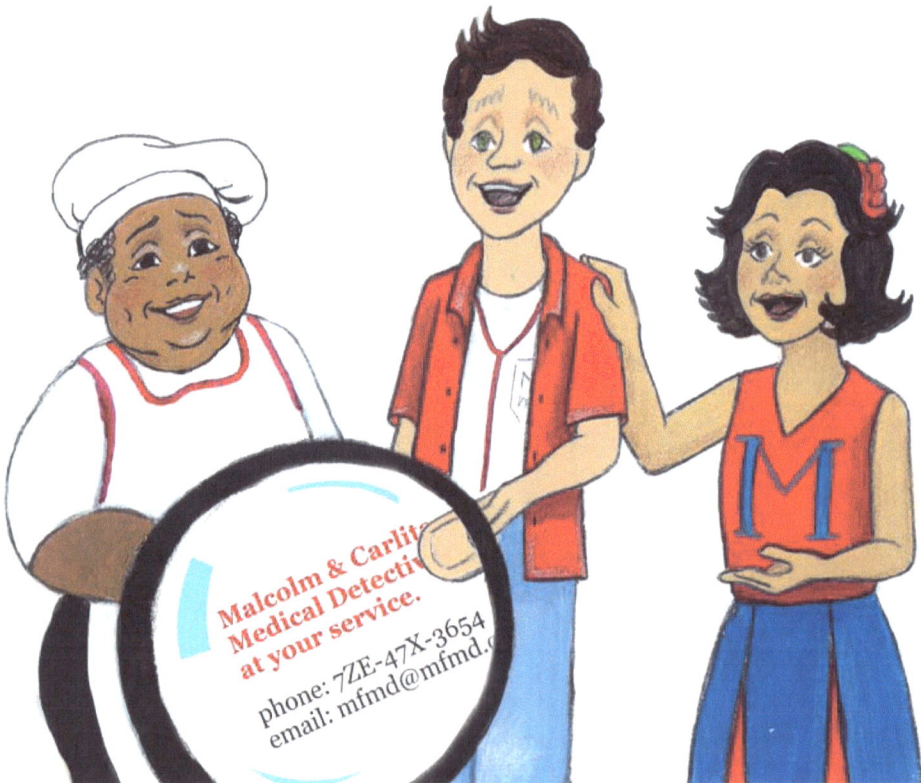

Malcolm & Carlita
Medical Detective
at your service.
phone: 7ZE-47X-3654
email: mfmd@mfmd.

"Fortunately I have **supplies in my backpack**," said Carlita. "Let's grab your measurements and make a few changes before the game resumes. Waist, chest, and head-to-toe. You're four feet five inches tall. I have just what we need: elastic bands in Boys – one size fits all. Over your shoulders and around your waist... and I need two more packages!"

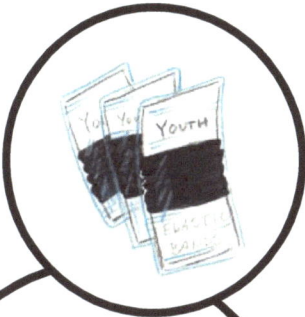

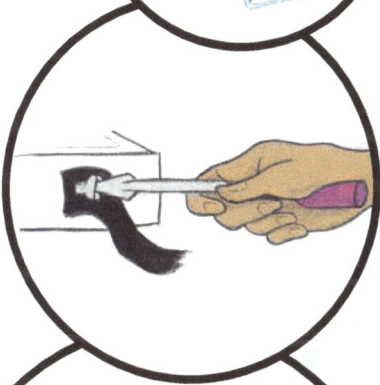

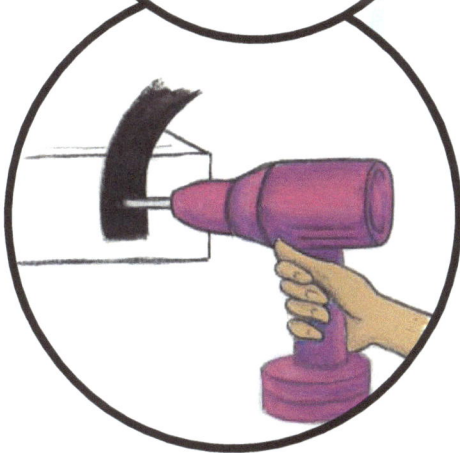

Good thing I have extras. A dab of glue, staples, screws..., and now you have a supportive tray.

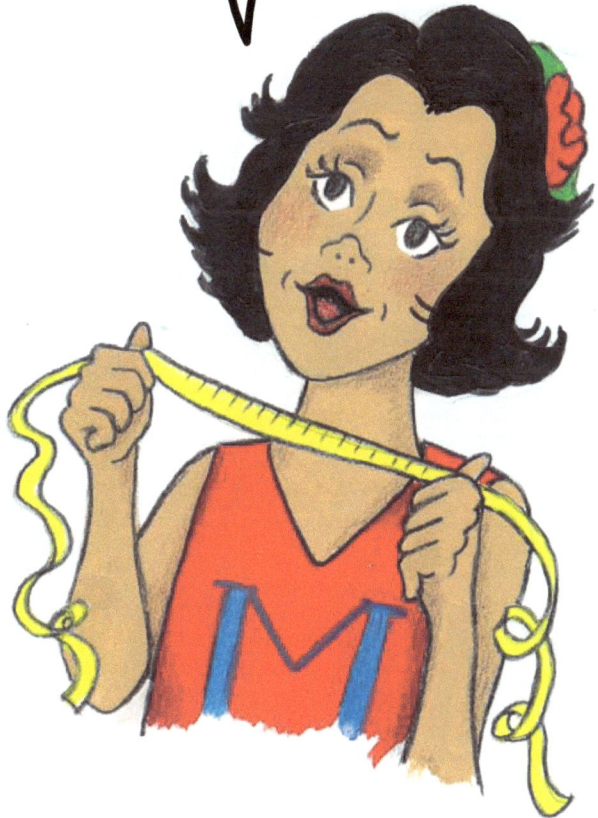

"Thanks to you two I'll be all set for the rest of the season and for this year's Ice Festival Competition," said Sugar. "Here are some brownies for all your hard work."

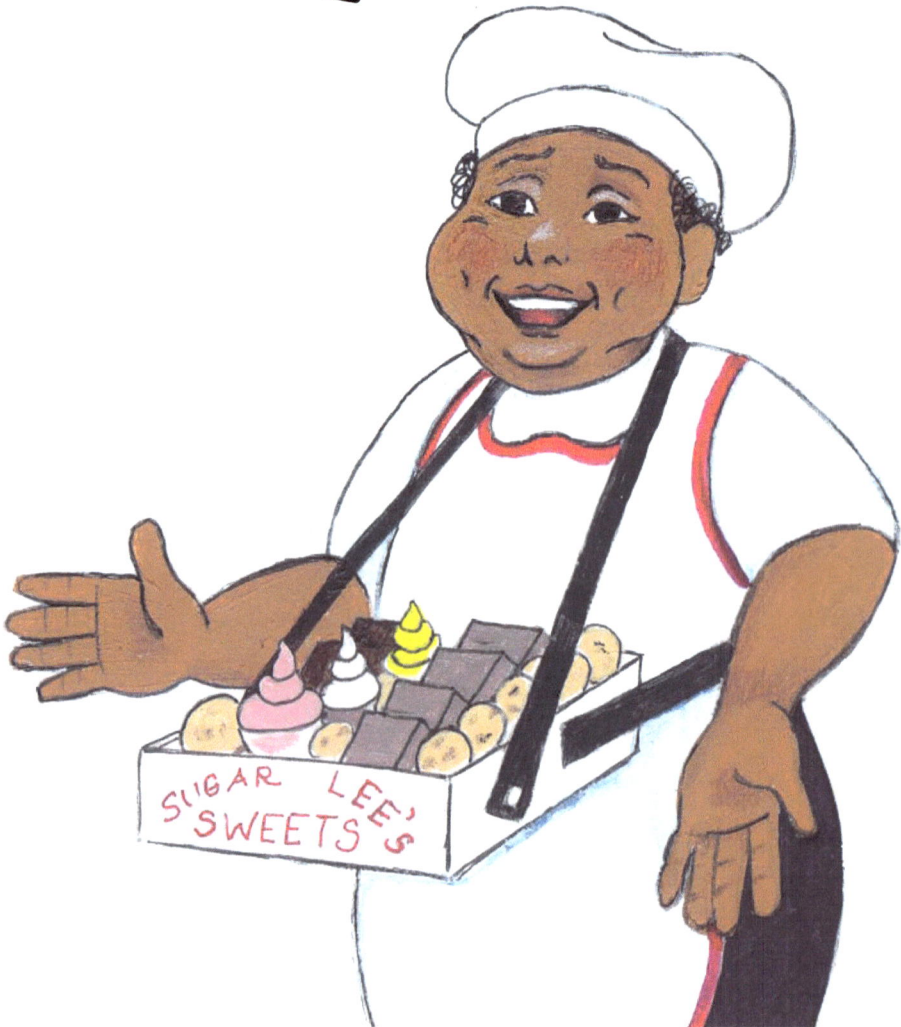

Carlita and Malcolm watched as Sugar began working the aisles. He reached and bent and ran from one customer to the next, weaving through the rows. As he reached the third aisle, beads of sweat rolled down his forehead. Then Malcolm and Carlita saw him plop down on the concrete steps.

"We have to help him!" said Malcolm. "What if he's having an asthma attack? The huffing and puffing with activity?"

"Well, we'd better get him to Milton Clinic," said Carlita. "Or at least back to headquarters to test our theories."

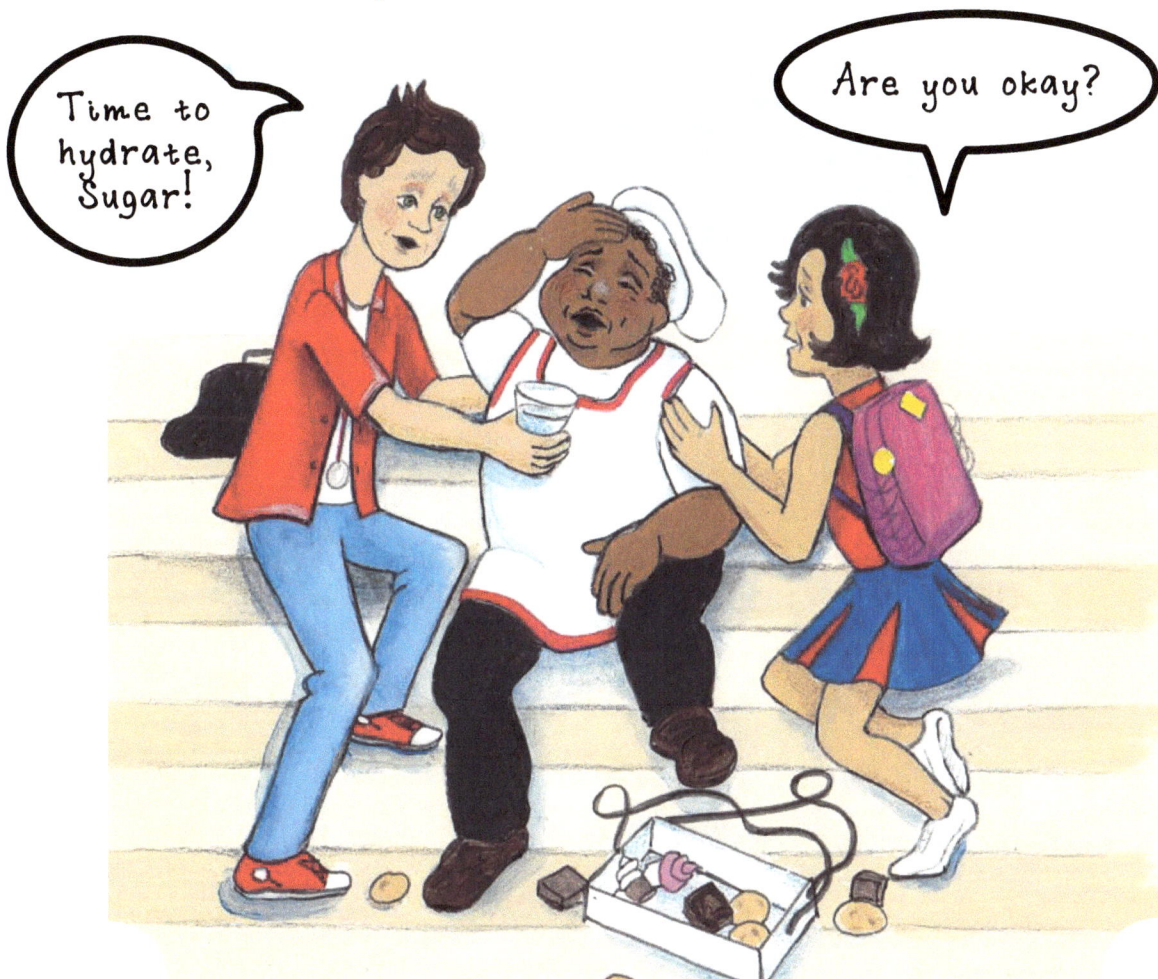

Back at Malcolm's attic headquarters, and after a few minutes of rest, Sugar looked better. He denied having asthma but Malcolm insisted that a complete investigation was necessary.

Let's get down to the lungs of this investigation. Tell me about the who, what, when, and where of your breathing problems.

Over the past few years, I've had a hard time breathing during activities. I get more tired and sweaty than other kids do.

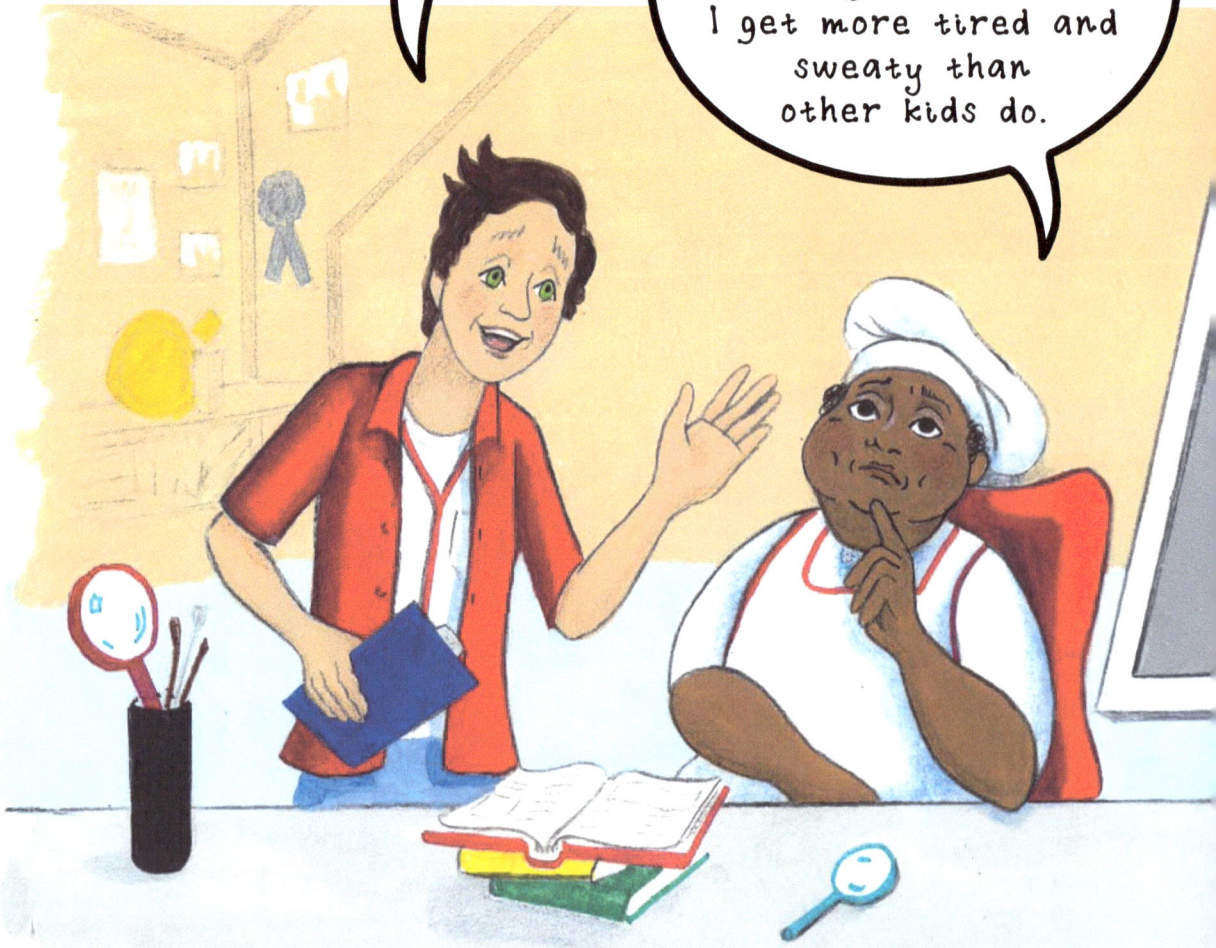

"Have you noticed any other strange symptoms?" asked Malcolm.

"I'm thirsty all the time," said Sugar. "I drink lots of soda, but then I have to take bathroom breaks a gazillion times a day. I also get monstrous belly grumbles. I'm too busy for meal breaks, so I load up on my own tasty treats."

Hmm. A few more questions, an exam, and we might have an answer.

SYMPTOMS:

1. REALLY THIRSTY

. EXTRA POTTY BREAKS

REALLY HUNGRY

DIFFICULTY BREATHING

EALLY TIRED. BEDTIME AT 8:00 PM

D WAKE TIME AT 7:00 AM TO BAKE

T AND SWEATY.

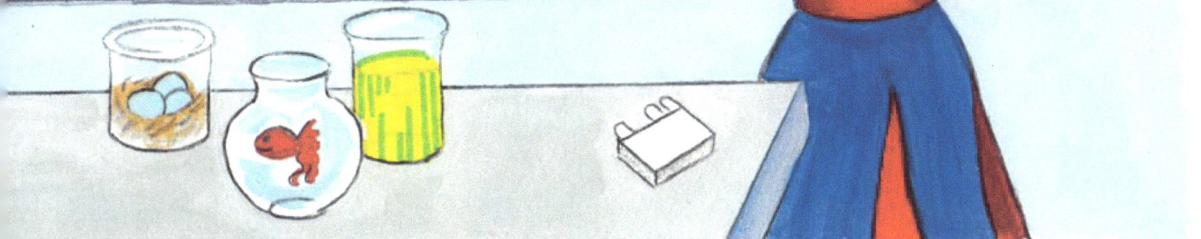

3. THE PHYSICAL EVIDENCE

Malcolm held up his stethoscope and listened to Sugar's chest and stomach. Carlita grabbed a machine with a big tube, cord, and lots of buttons and set it in front of Malcolm.

"Spirometer ready," said Carlita. "So what's the diagnosis so far? Could it be…?"

"Well, no lung harmonicas; they sound as clear as an ocean breeze," interrupted Malcolm. "Now let's check your lung strength."

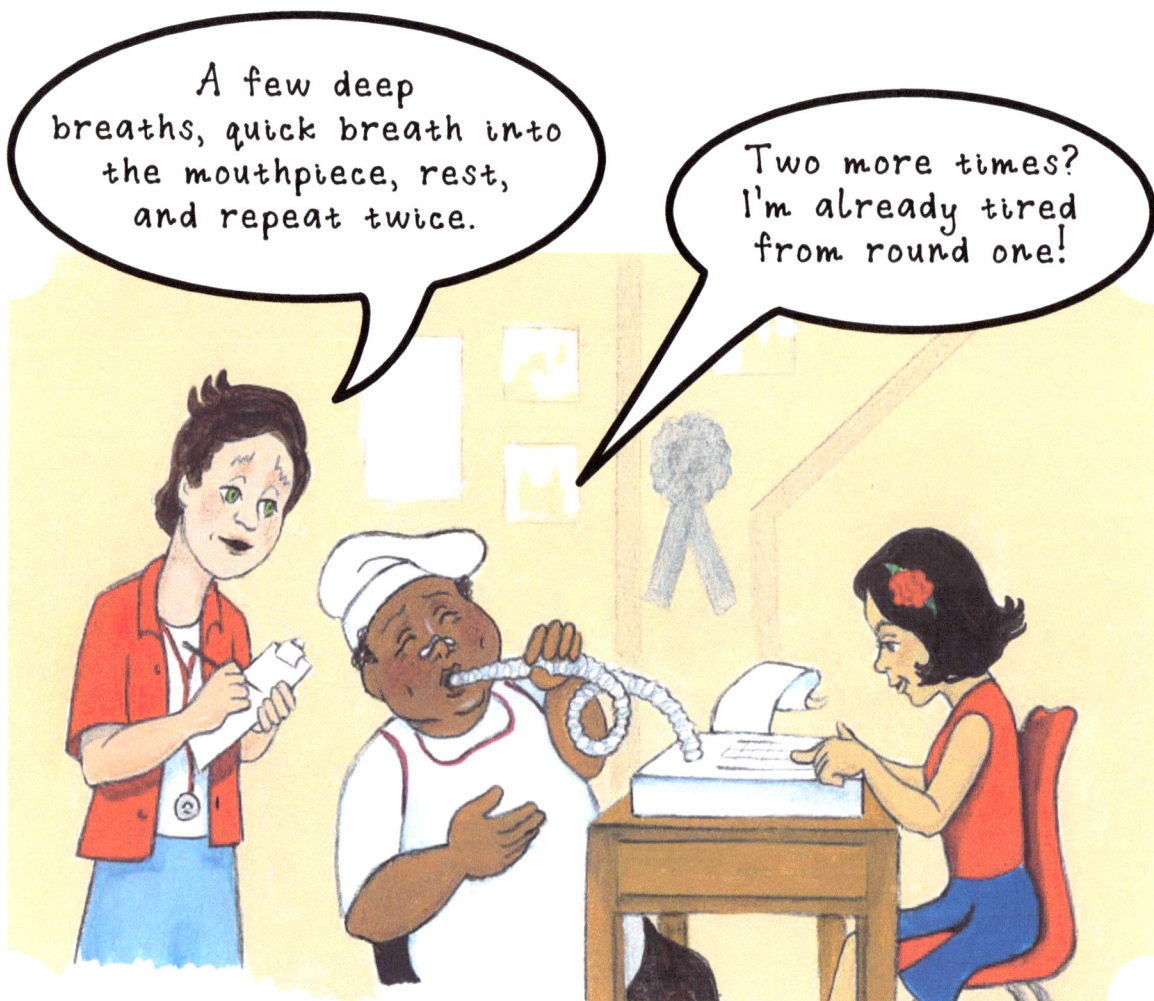

A few deep breaths, quick breath into the mouthpiece, rest, and repeat twice.

Two more times? I'm already tired from round one!

When Sugar finished the test, Carlita handed the results to Malcolm.

"Your numbers show lung strength as powerful as other kids your age," said Malcolm. "But I have one last test. Genome, come here, little guy."

Genome padded into the room, Malcolm tossed him into Sugar's arms, ruffled the cat's fur and sent strands flying into the air.

I love animals.

Ah-choo. I don't think he has allergies Malcolm but what about...

Touché Carlita. No asthma or allergies like you, but we're still missing something.

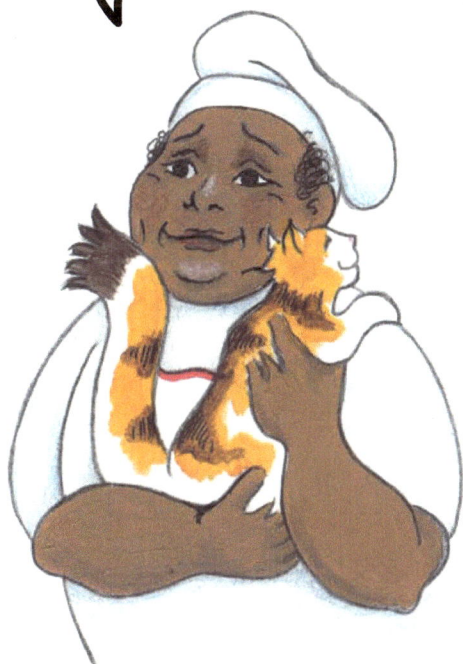

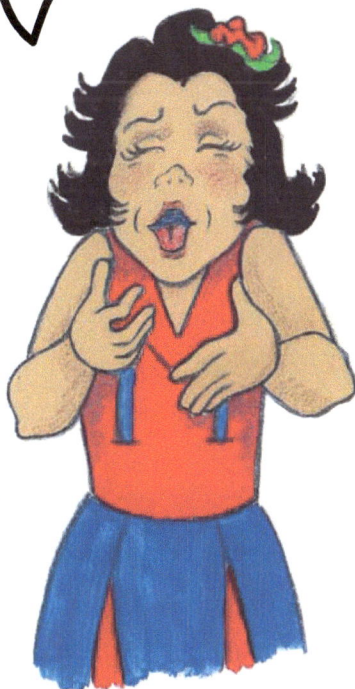

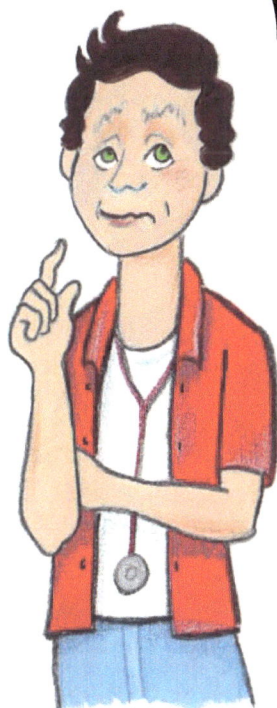

Carlita snapped her fingers at Malcolm. She stepped behind Sugar and disappeared, then stepped out again.

"Do you see?" said Carlita. "The clue you're missing is right in front of you. Sugar is a great baker, a good business kid, and has a great pair of lungs. But...really look at the big picture Malcolm."

"Criminy Cardiac!" exclaimed Malcolm. "Well, uh, Sugar? Has anyone ever mentioned that you may be a little bigger than most kids your age?"

There's more to this than just baby fat. Time for a frosty trudge to the science museum secret laboratory.

My momma always says this is baby fat, just like my brothers had.

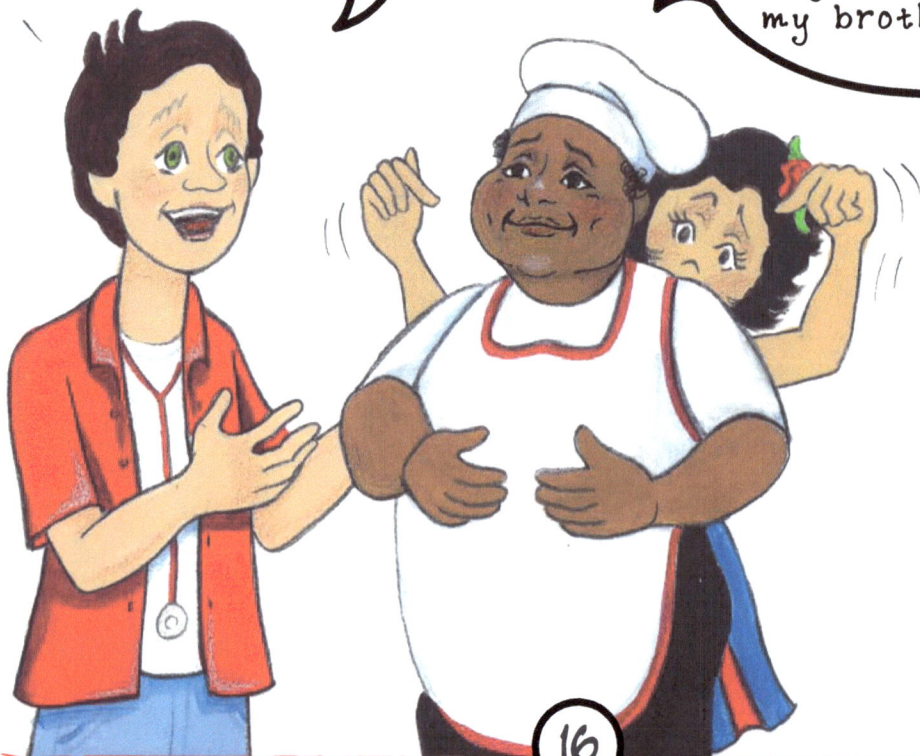

At the museum, Malcolm escorted his friends to an office. The sign on the door read, "Mr. Finney, Chief Invention Coordinator." As Malcolm grabbed a set of keys, his dad turned around.

"Hey there! Solving another medical mystery I see," said Mr. Finney. "I stored an amazing new invention in the 'Mad Scientists Laboratory'. It's a time machine! I haven't quite worked out all the kinks, but NEATO, RIGHT!?"

"Very neat! See you later, Dad," said Malcolm.

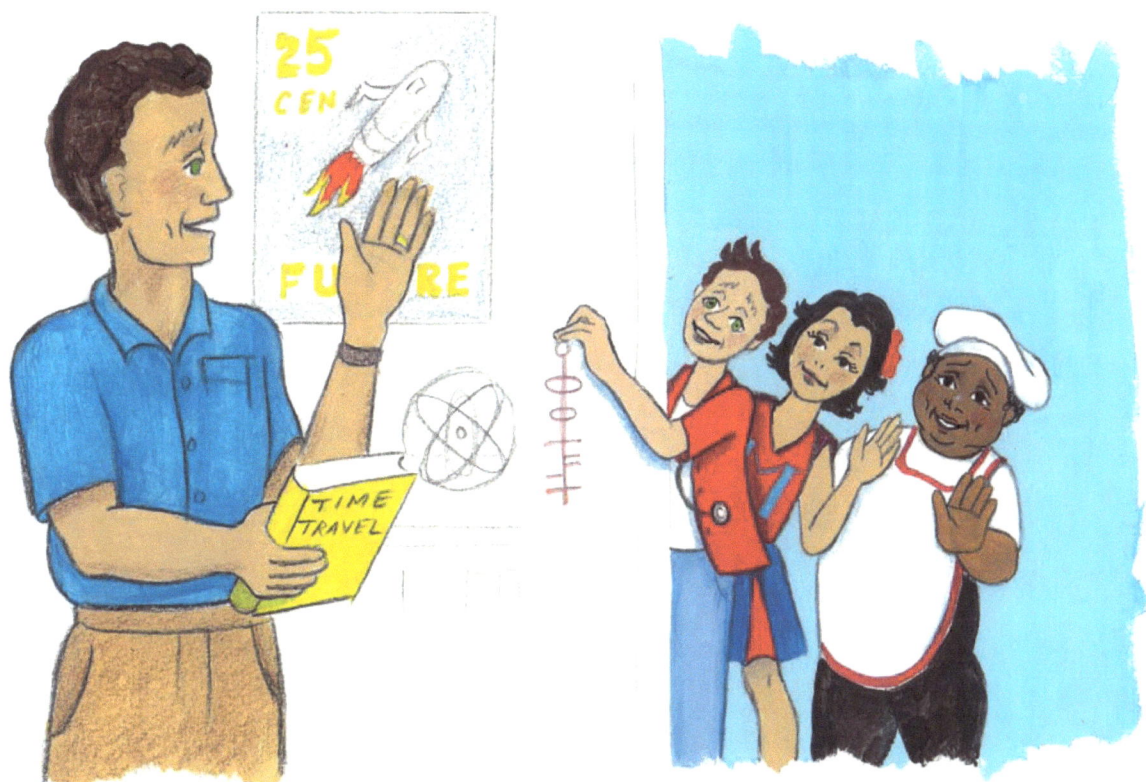

"My partner was right in thinking your size could be a problem. Let's weigh you and crunch some numbers," said Malcolm.

"Scale ready," said Carlita. "Up you go Sugar. One hundred and thirty pounds. So we put this number, along with your height, into our computer for a nine-year-old and…. your BMI is…"

BMI (Body Mass Index):

A calculated number that helps measure body fat.

32! That's over the 95th percentile, which means you're carrying more weight than 95 percent of kids your age. It means you're obese!

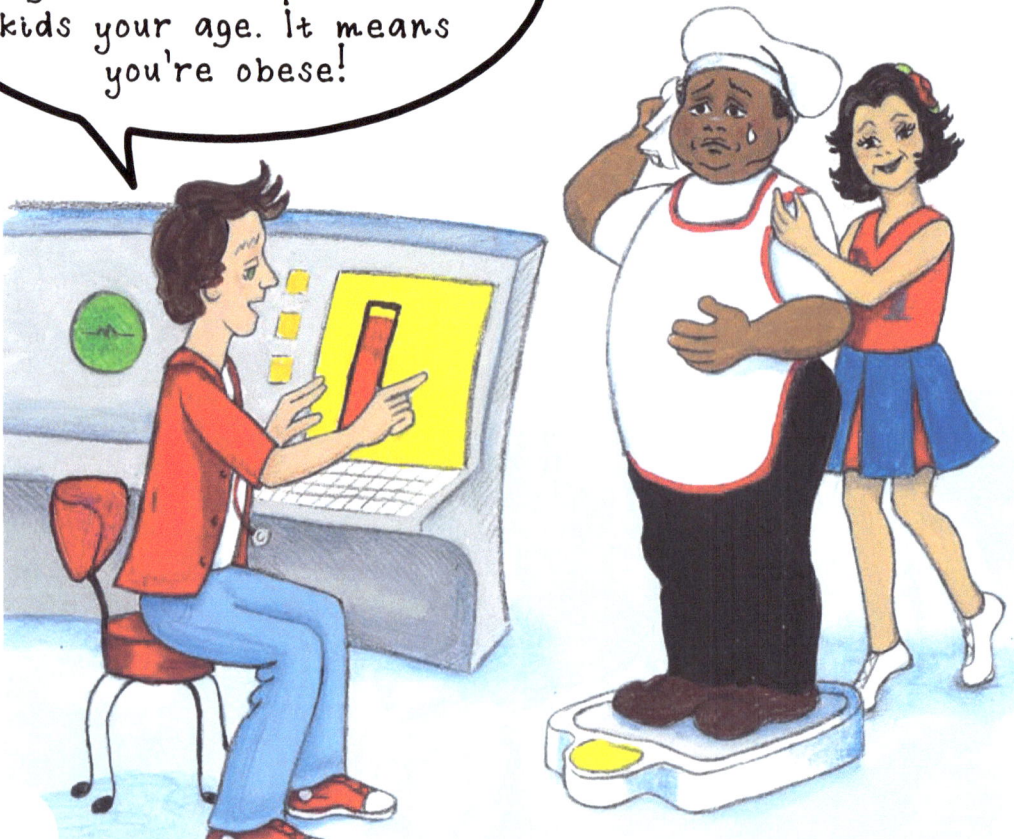

4. THE INVESTIGATION

After Carlita calmed Sugar, Malcolm sprayed everyone down with a protective skin coating. Sugar climbed into the tank of Intelli-Goo. Laser light moved across the goo tank.

This is starting to look like a Frankenstein movie. I'd better come out of here the same as I went in.

Besides the stitches in your scalp, where I removed your brain and replaced it with another one, right? Just kidding.

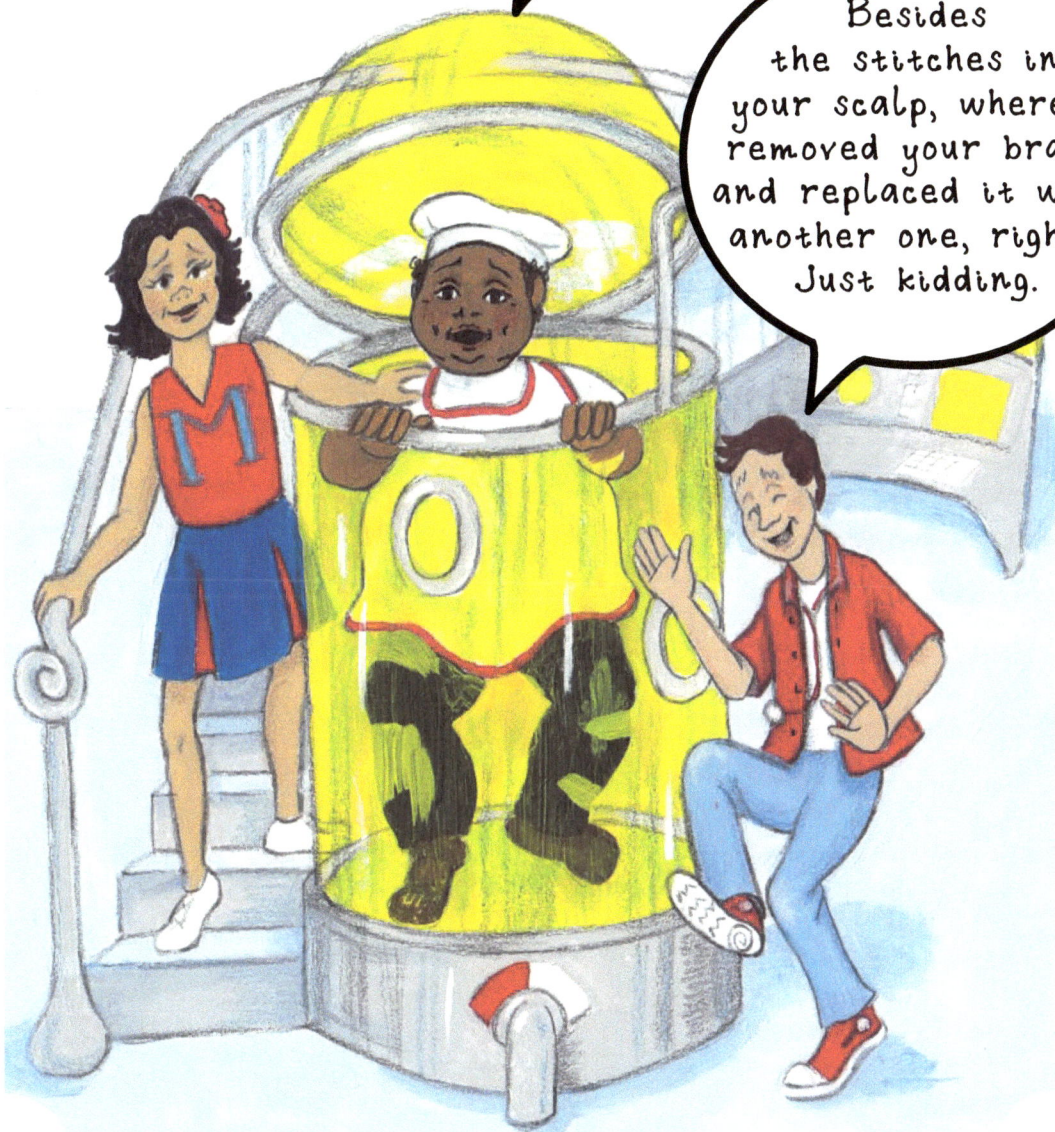

Malcolm slapped wrist-walkies on Sugar and Carlita. He told the computer to create interactive lungs and an abdomen. Intelli-Goo started spilling onto the floor. Walls of yellow, jiggly blocks popped up all around and underneath the trio. Soon they were wedged between the blocks.

"Help! I'm stuck," shouted Carlita. "Now I can imagine how you feel, Sugar. Fat tissue can be really... heavy, especially if it's sitting... on... your... chest."

"Exactamundo!" said Malcolm. "You've found the first clue. We know that Sugar's lungs can work normally, but the fat pressure makes it a difficult job. "

It's so heavy...I... I can't breathe.

Hang in there! You're one big tug away from fresh air.

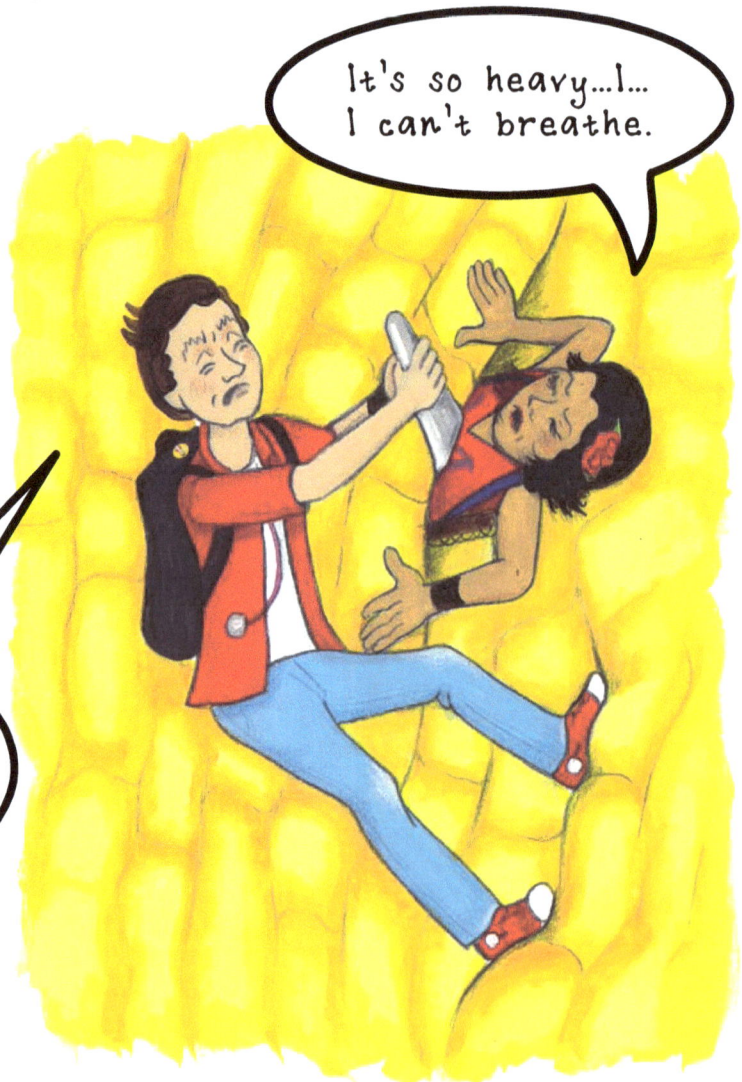

After freeing Carlita, Malcolm continued tunneling through the fat layer until he saw what looked like mounds of giant pink worms. He connected everyone to a rope, grabbed a reflex hammer for climbing, and stopped in front of a pink crescent-shaped organ.

"Phew!" said Sugar. "I'm glad we're out of that smelly area. That was like climbing over a garbage dump."

"It's the smell of your lunch gurgling through the intestines," said Malcolm. "But we've reached our destination, the stomach."

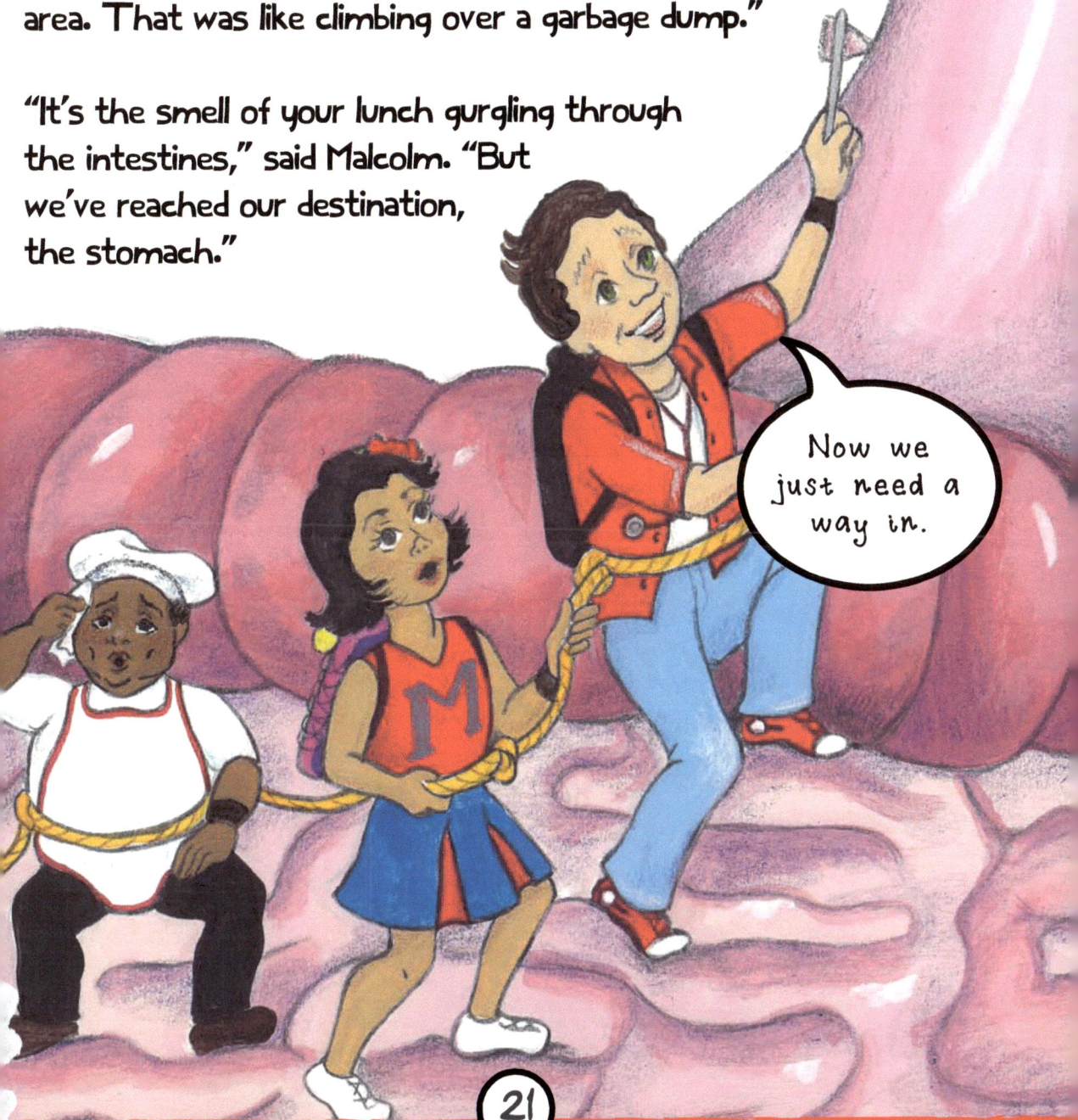

Now we just need a way in.

Carlita pulled a contraption from her bag and fired it at the stomach. *Click…click…click.* The plunger rotated on the stomach wall. **Zzzzzzzip!** A cord retracted, creating an entrance.

As the trio stepped into the gum colored-organ, a rocking motion churned them over a patch of wavy grooves.

"Cookies again?" asked Malcolm. "

"Um," said Sugar. "It was a busy day. I forgot my lunch."

"Whoa!" said Carlita. "That liquid is melting the food like heat on plastic. I'm scared!"

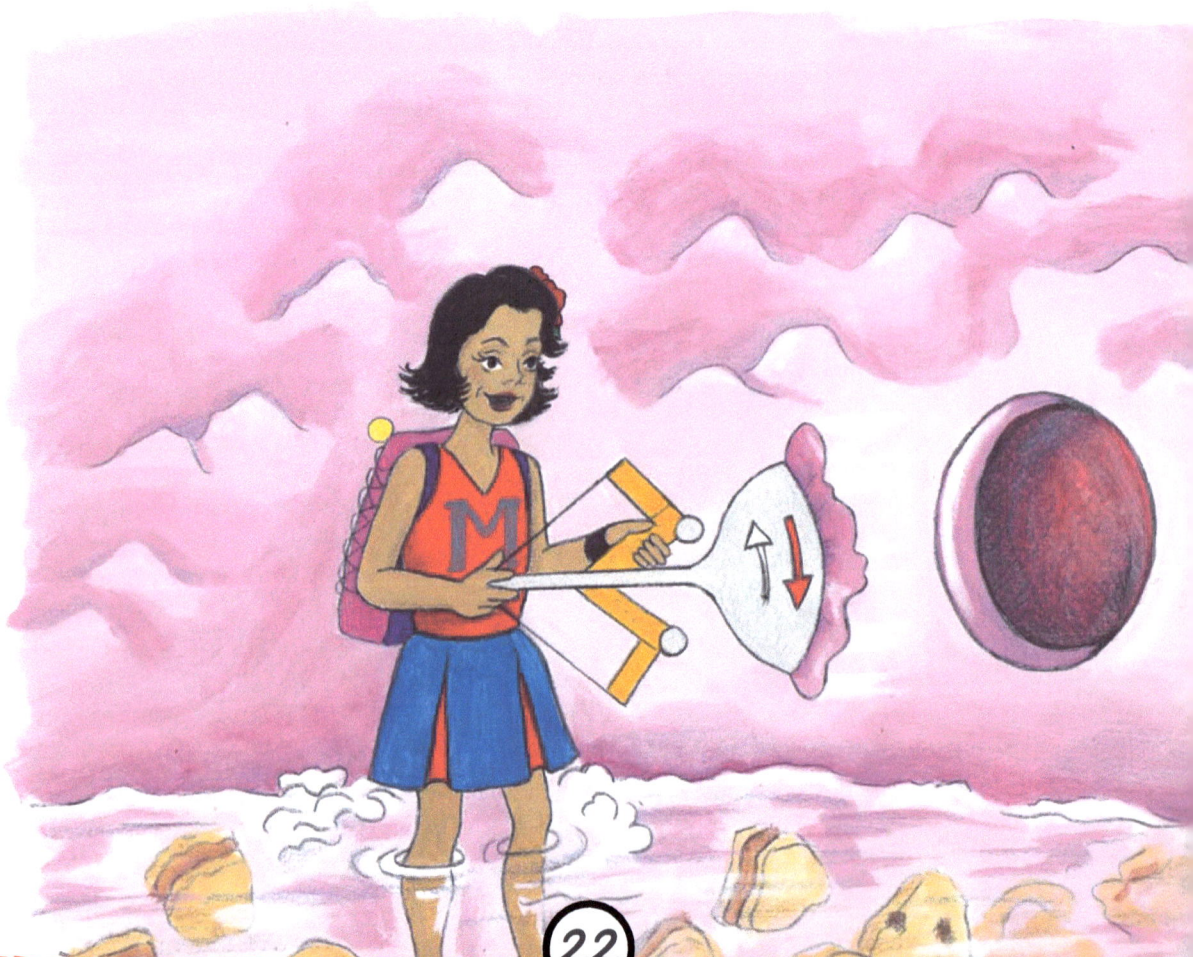

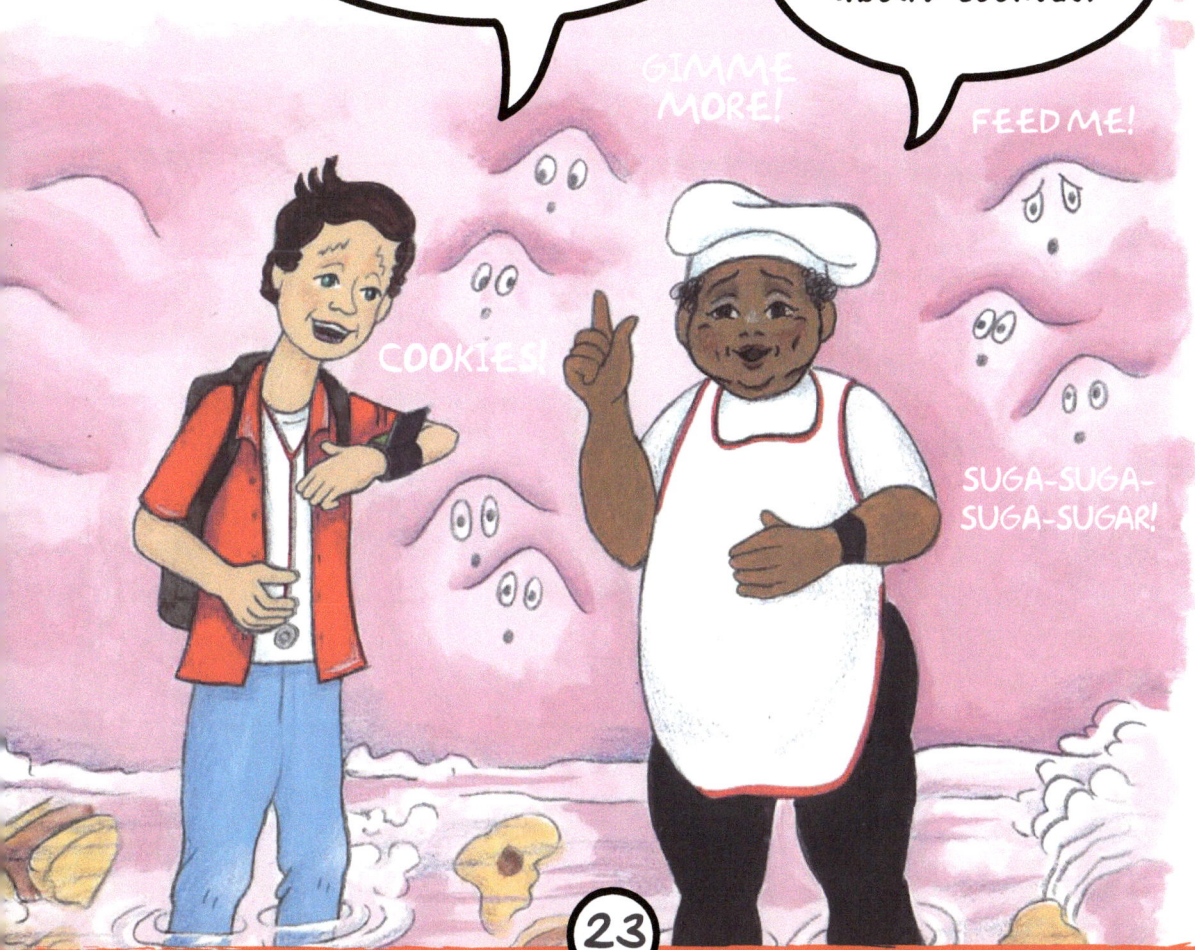

Amidst the noise, the stomach exit opened. The cookie goop sloshed between the cells on its way out. The stomach cells stopped their cookie discussion and began a chorus of noises.

Carlita, Malcolm, and Sugar splurted through the pyloric sphincter and into the small intestines.

The small intestines release chemicals that break up food and transport nutrients, before sending it to the colon for dumping.

I'm up here... getting seasick!

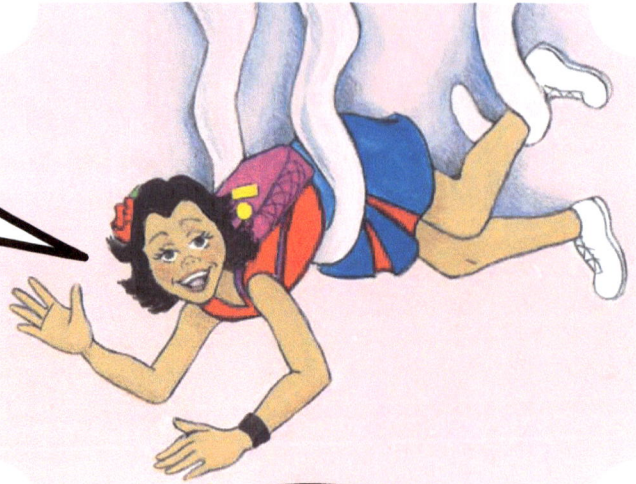

These swaying shag-like fronds are villi. They're like sponges that absorb nutrients. Hey, where's Carlita?

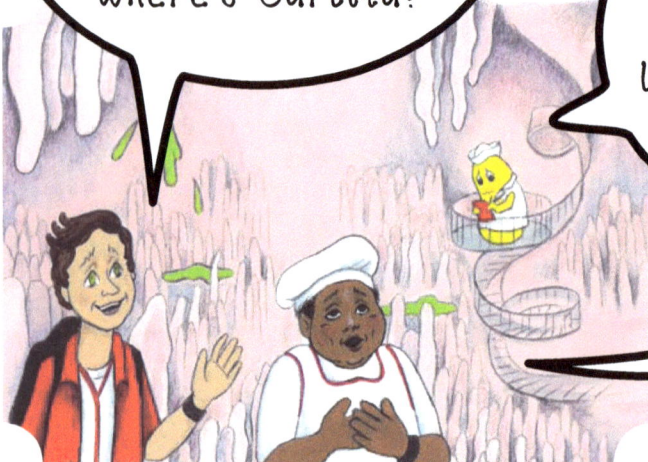

What do we have here? A little fat, some sugar. Looks like we need more insulin... like always!

Shag carpet walls and floors?

After untangling Carlita the group ran to the tower and down the stairs just in time to see the messenger boating away. Malcolm dug in his medical bag and pulled out a folded-up rubber canoe. He threw a pair of expandable paddles to Carlita and Sugar.

"Follow him," said Malcolm. "Time for a visit to the Islets of Langerhans, in pancreatic country. That's where insulin is made. It may be the source of this problem."

It was smooth paddling up the capillary until the blood vessel widened and the canoe began to move faster.

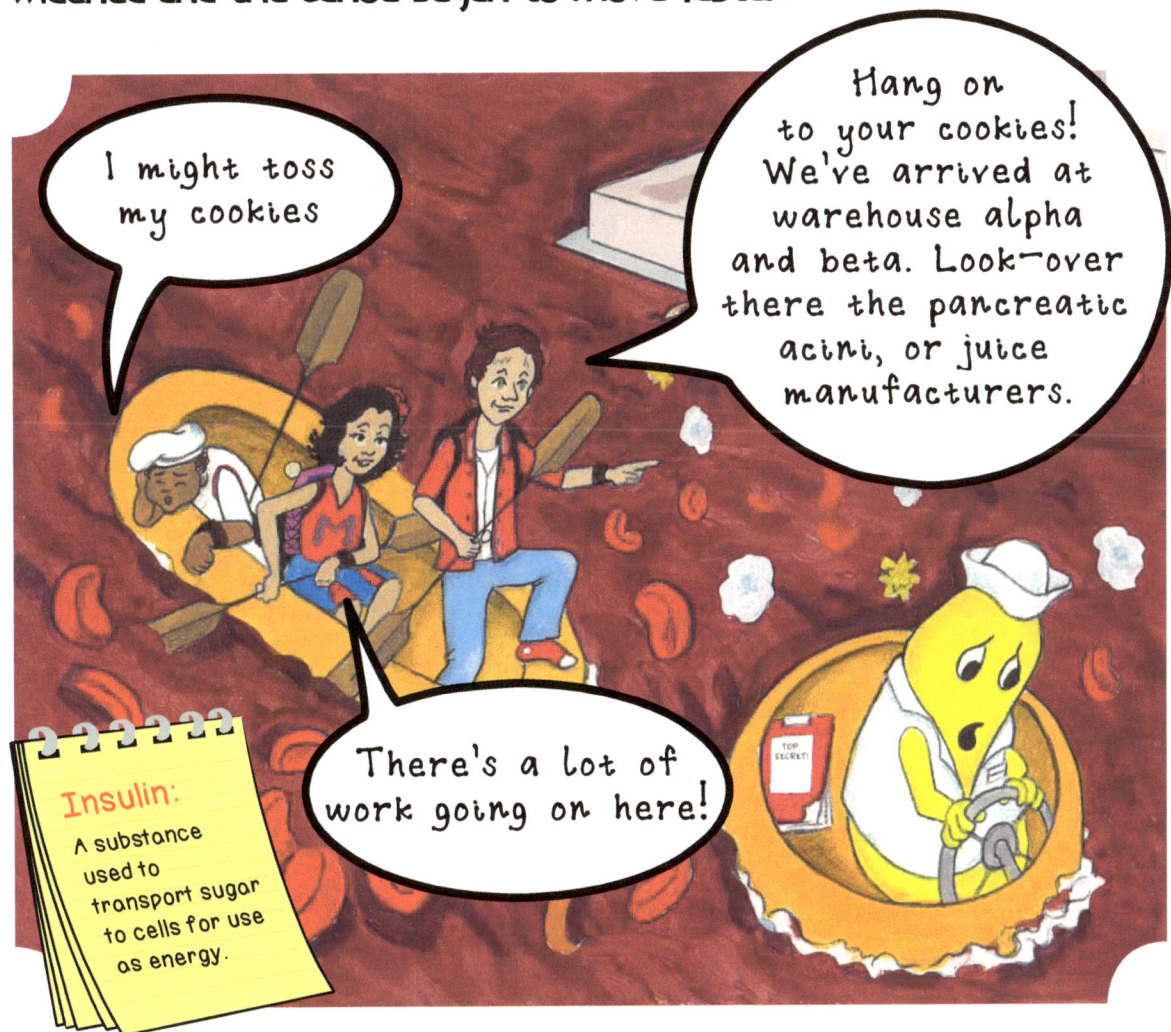

I might toss my cookies

Hang on to your cookies! We've arrived at warehouse alpha and beta. Look-over there the pancreatic acini, or juice manufacturers.

There's a lot of work going on here!

Insulin:
A substance used to transport sugar to cells for use as energy.

"The pancreas is quite a factory," said Malcolm. "The beta cells make the hormone insulin to unlock tissues like the fat, muscle, and liver so they can take in glucose for energy. Insulin also advises cells to stop using stored energy and switch to energy from digested food. The acini cells make those juices that just sprayed us in the small intestines to digest food. Cool, huh?"

"It's a marvelous invention," said Carlita. "Hey, it looks like those hormones are catching and counting glucose."

As the group paddled closer, they could hear Supervisor Sam Insulin and Assistant Manager Henry Insulin arguing.

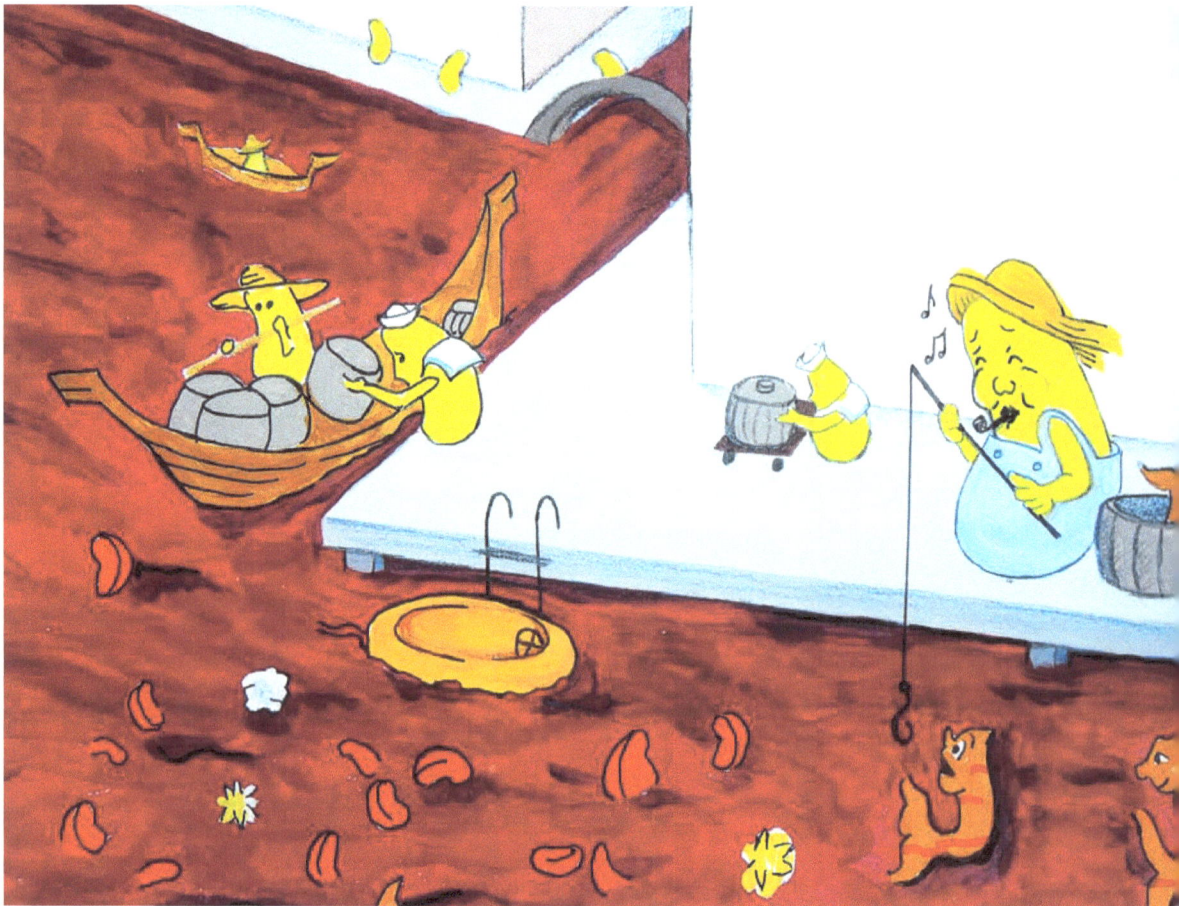

"Okay, men," said Supervisor Sam Insulin. "We're over-flooded with glucose and we need to sell these before the supply goes stale. If we let these critters keep swimming free, they'll wreak havoc on our river systems and our wallets."

"But, sir," said Assistant Manager Henry Insulin. "The communities insist they have too much already. They refuse to open their doors or unlock their pantries or gates."

"No excuses!" yelled Supervisor Sam Insulin. "If you can't get the liver or muscle cells to open up, then offer it to the fat cells. They always take extra glucose. If all else fails, use your master key."

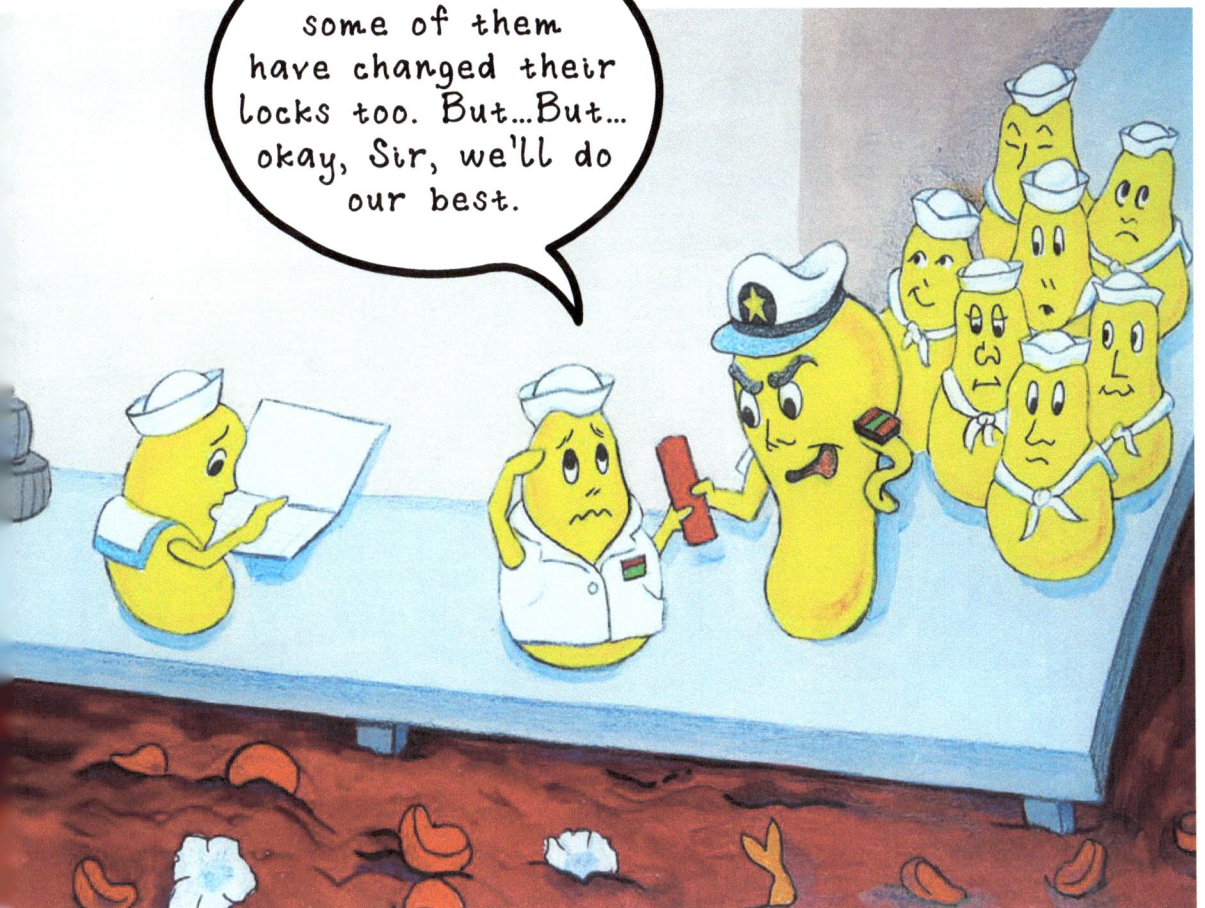

But Sir, some of them have changed their locks too. But...But... okay, Sir, we'll do our best.

5. THE DX

"Criminy Cardiac!" exclaimed Malcolm. "That's it. The cells are resisting the insulin salesmen because they already have too much glucose. The fat cells can take some because of their storage duties, even if they have to create new fat cells for the excess. But large amounts of glucose still circulate in the vessel-rivers, unable to be stored or used, which is called... DIABETES! Now, there are a few more things we need to figure this out in the laboratory.

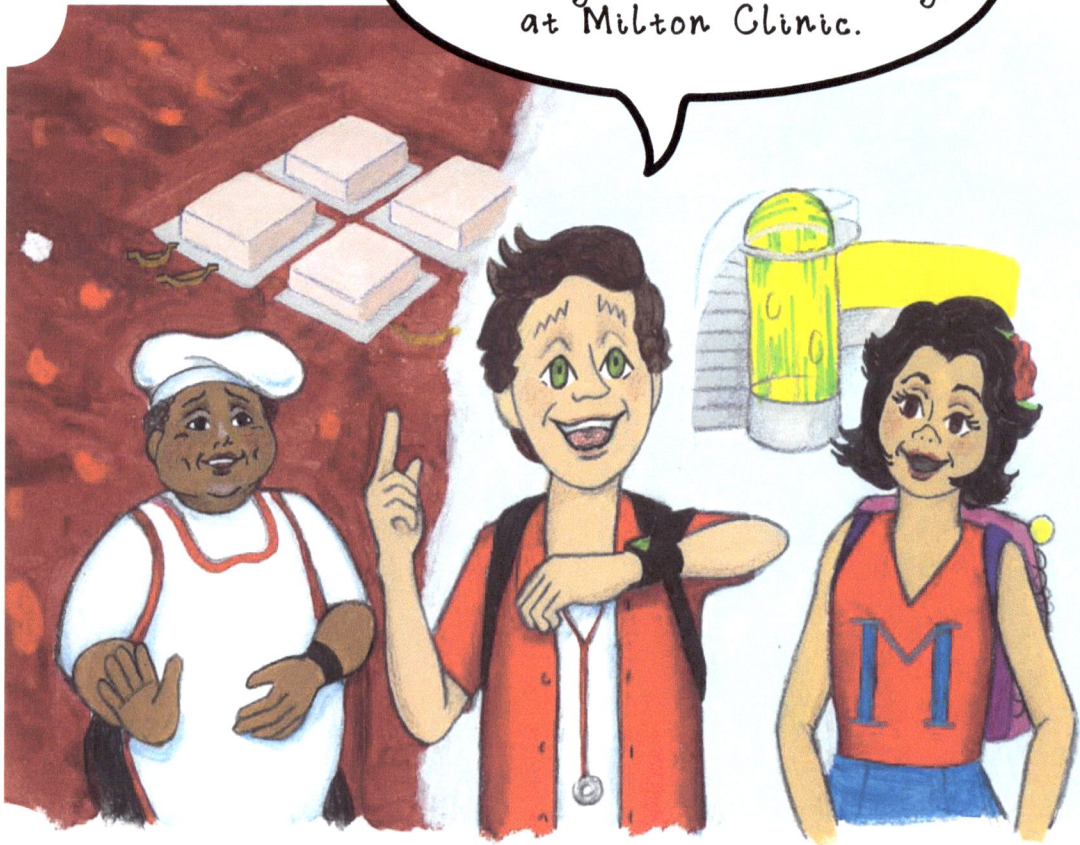

Exit interactive animation. It's time to visit my mom, Dr. Finney, at Milton Clinic.

"Diabetes is a likely explanation for what you saw," said Mrs. Finney. "Let's measure Sugar's sugar. Two hundred! Normal is below 100. We'll have to do more tests, a physical exam, and discuss concerns with Sugar's parents. In the meantime, you two teach Sugar how a healthy body is made."

"Got it covered," said Malcolm. "We'll start working on his body care guide and have it ready by tomorrow."

"I don't think so, Malcolm," said Sugar. "I can move my fingers, legs, and toes. That's all I really need to be a great baker. My momma and my family are big-boned just like me. Thanks for your help, but I have a busy night of baking ahead."

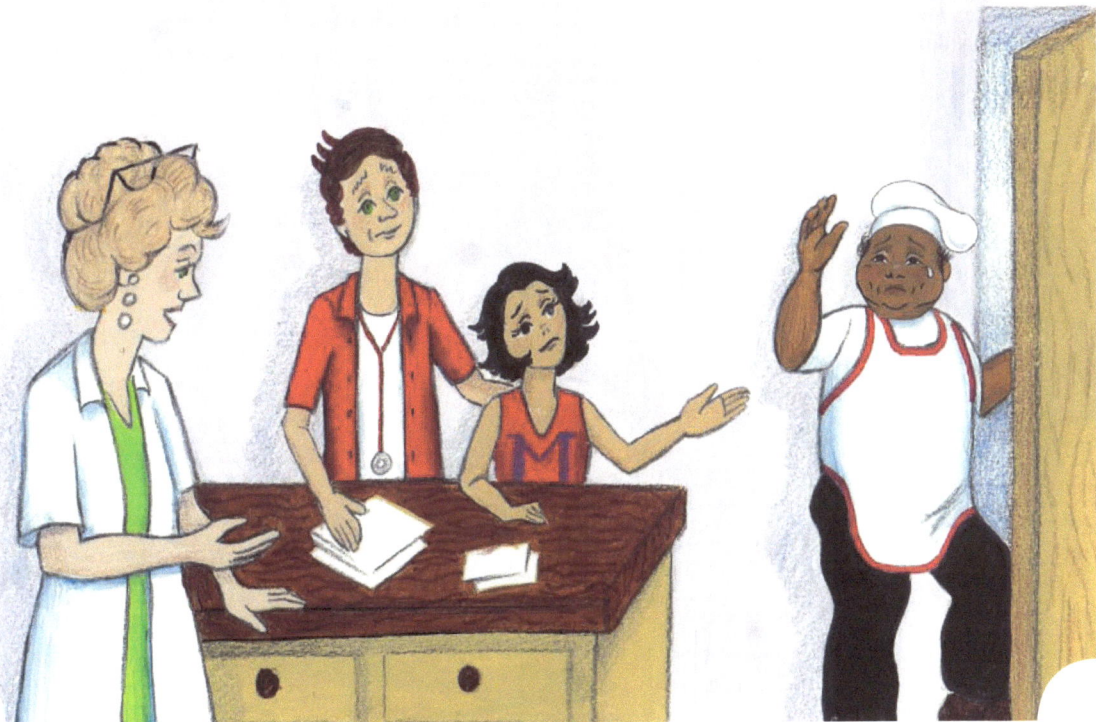

Malcolm and Carlita headed back to the attic office and slumped in front of the TV. Malcolm hung his head and sighed.

"He doesn't realize how this will affect his life," said Carlita. "Don't let it get you down, it's the holidays. Besides, one of my favorite movies is on: A Christmas Carol."

"Carlita That's IT!" said Malcolm. "Genius! He doesn't understand how becoming obese can affect his life now or later. Unless...he can see it first-hand. I hope you can operate the time machine. I have a plan."

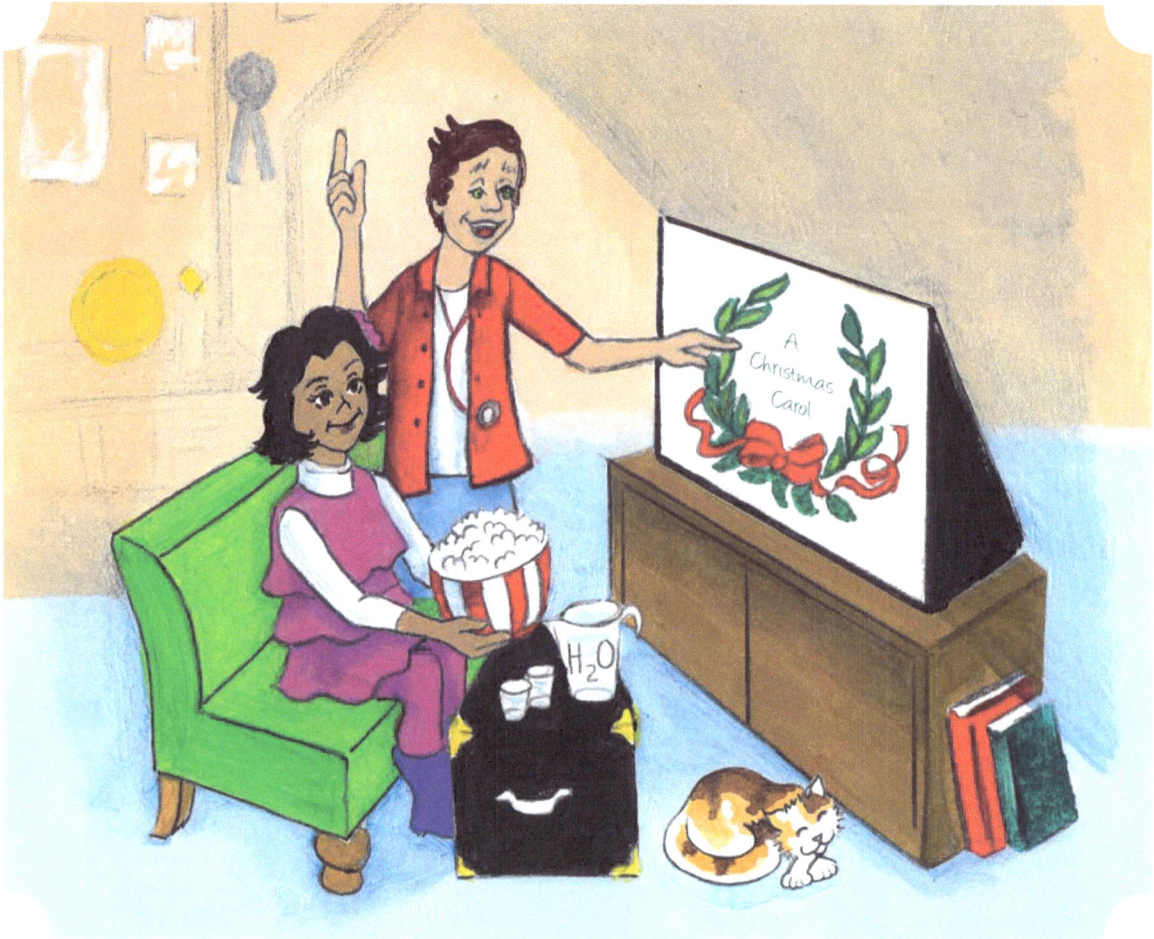

By the time they had gathered their supplies and constructed their costumes, it was sundown. Malcolm, Carlita, and Genome connected their sled to a snowmobile and slid over to Sugar's house.

"The window's open," said Malcolm. "I'll climb through, and you hold the ladder. Let the mission begin."

"Make it quick," said Carlita. "Genome isn't your typical guard dog, uh, or guard ghost."

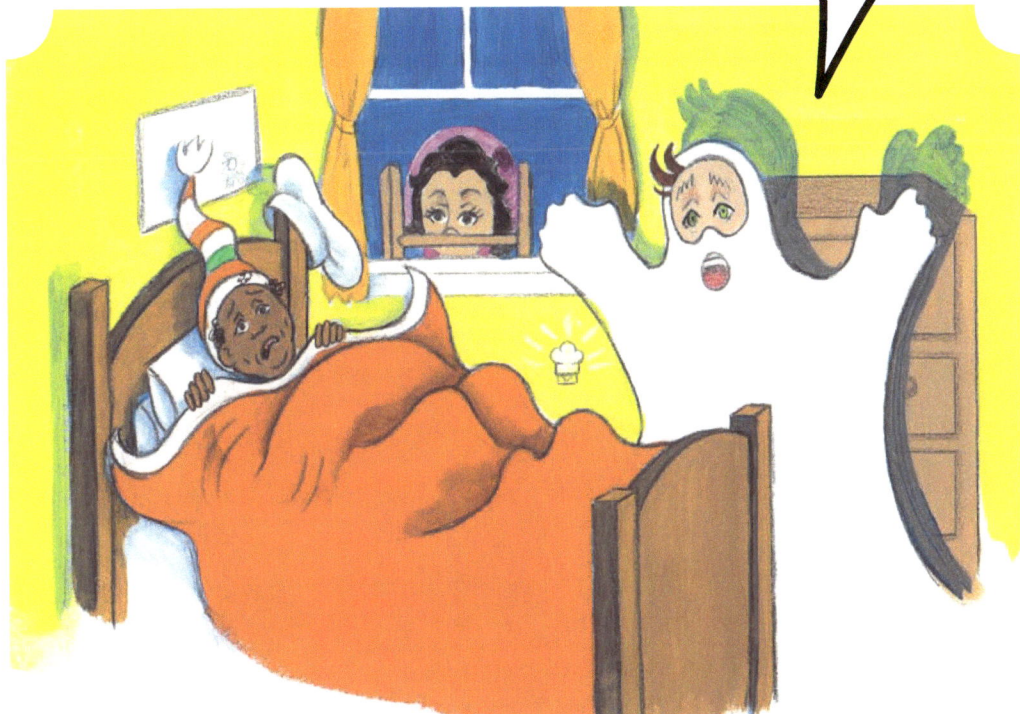

Wooo...Woooo... Wooooo. Wake up, Sugar Lee. I am your ghost guide, here to take you on a health journey this cold winter's night. Let us see your road to obesity and diabetes. Come with me.

After boarding the snowmobile, the trio made their way back to Malcolm's secret laboratory. They strapped themselves into the time machine and Carlita set it to Sugar's first year of life. After a splatter of light, a whirl, and a whiz, they found themselves sitting in front of a baby Sugar.

"My favorite kiddie meal!" said Sugar. "Nuggets, French fries, and juice. Chicken and juice are good for you right? You got me on the fries, but we only had fast food a few times a week."

"Wooo-Wooo," howled Malcolm. "A healthy meal can be reversed just by unhealthy preparation. Grill instead of fry, whole fruit instead of juice, and add a heaping helping of steamed veggies."

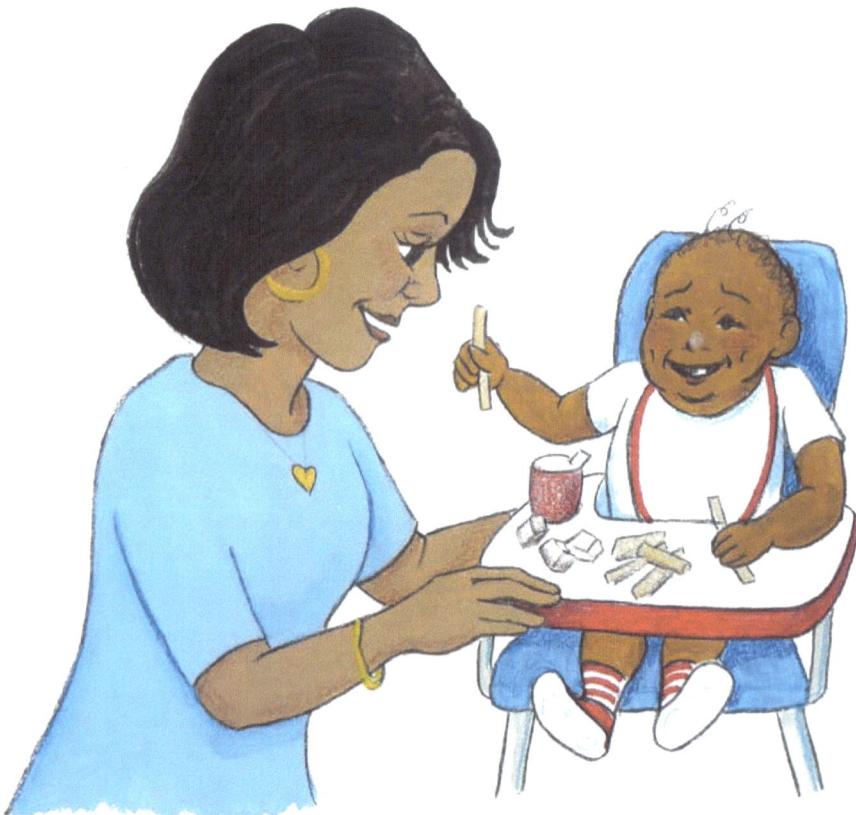

Malcolm whispered to Carlita to fast-forward through a few years. The time machine slowly clicked past scenes in Sugar's life.

"You ate a lot of unhealthy snacks" said Malcolm. "Not a fruit or glass of milk in sight. Ohhh, Ohhhh, Ohhhhh."

"You are a dramatic ghost," said Sugar. "Look! It's my junior football team with Daddy coaching. I was a little man full of energy. I didn't get pudgy until I stopped playing and started baking. Sharing sweet surprises with Momma always brought a smile to her face. It made me want to be a baker."

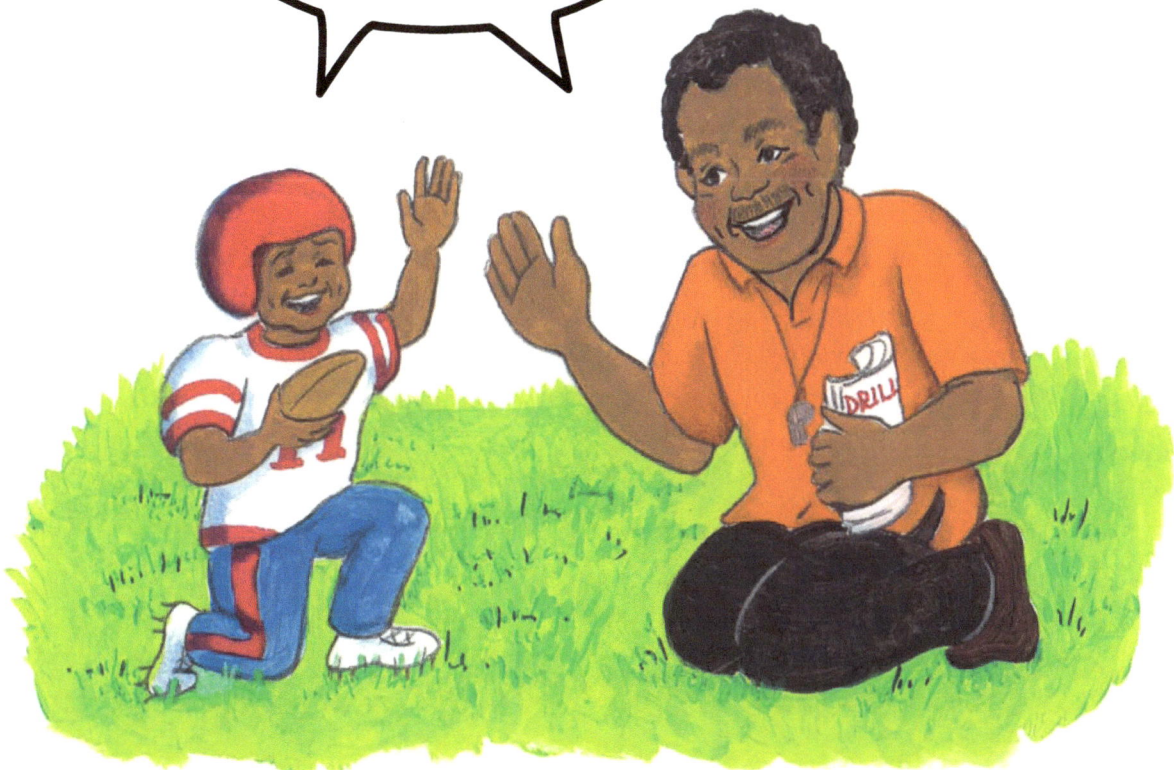

HIGH FIVE!

The time machine sped ahead to a young Sugar enjoying his favorite pastime.

"Wow," said Sugar. "Looks like Momma got plumper too. She worked a lot and our family began eating fast food more. I started baking daily pastries for the family."

"You show your love for people by offering them baked gifts, which makes them feel good," said Carlita. "But that feeling can be short-lived and the negative physical effects long-lasting. Let's see what happened after a few years of sugary gift giving."

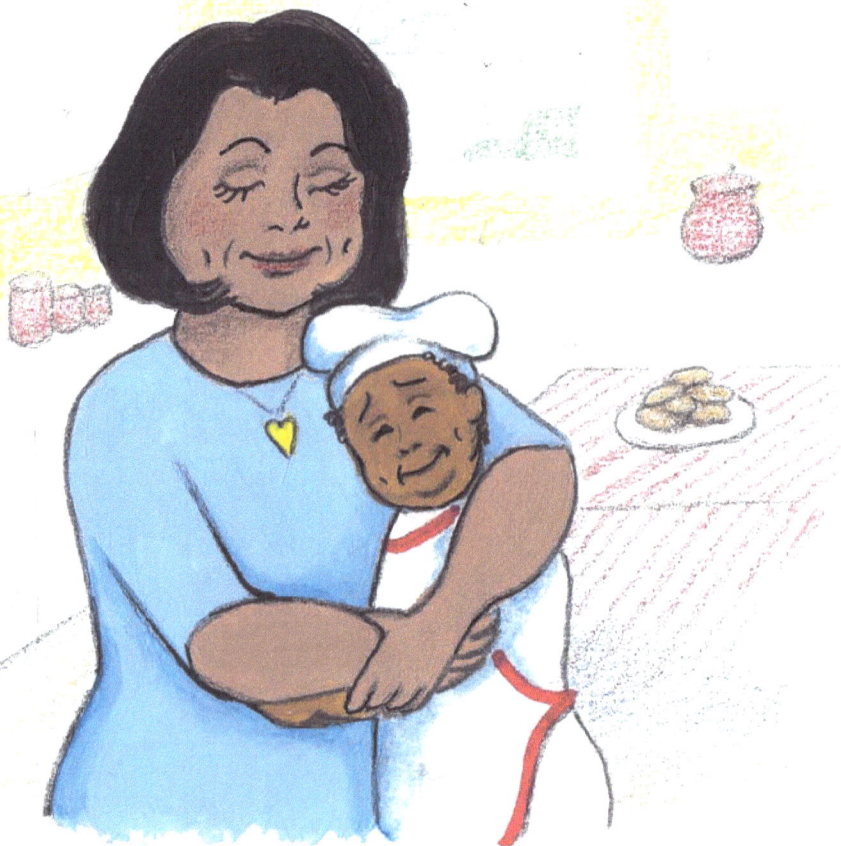

Carlita snapped the time machine into future mode. The group zipped away and landed in a hospital supply room. Malcolm handed everyone a pair of scrubs. He sent Genome to check if the coast was clear. After a furry nod and meow, Malcolm wheeled Sugar on a gurney to room 126 and closed the curtain. Before Malcolm could explain, someone walked in to see Sugar's roommate.

"Mr. Lee Jones, or Sugar as you're called, I'm Doctor Wald. I'm sorry to say we can't save your toe. This diabetes is out of control, making your blood ripe for an infection like gangrene."

After we remove it, we can discuss how to get you healthy and moving again.

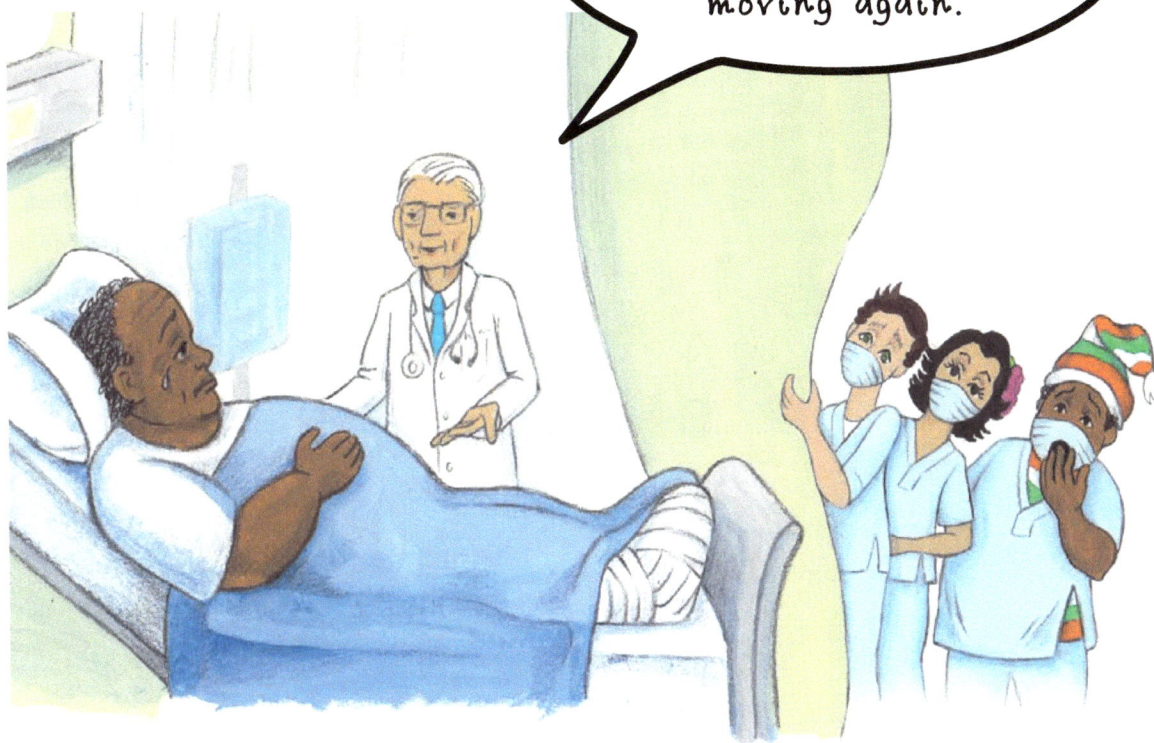

Doctor Wald closed the curtain and left the room.

"That's me!" said Sugar. "They're gonna take my big toe! And I can't even walk. That means I can't bake anymore. No way! This will not happen."

Two nurses opened Sugar's curtain and stood at his bedside. "Okay, Lee," said the nurses. "We're here to take you to surgery." They began pushing Sugar's bed out of the room. Malcolm and Carlita jumped up.

"Wait, wait!" screamed Carlita. "You've got the wrong Lee."

"Carlita, get the time machine ready," said Malcolm. "We'll meet you there."

"Yeah. I'm not Mr. Jones," said Sugar. "I mean I am, but I'm not."

OH NO! YOU CAN'T TAKE MY BIG TOE!

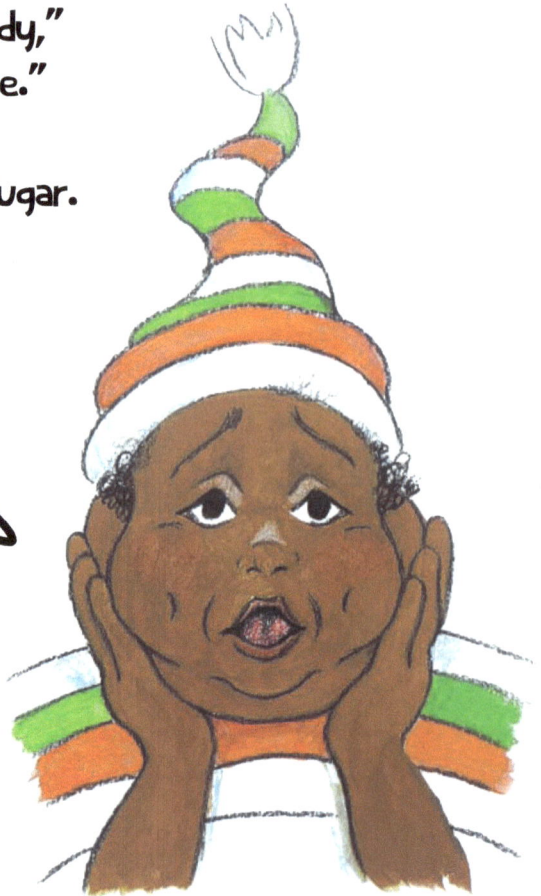

Malcolm grabbed the front of the gurney from the nurses, swung right and ran toward the supply room, where Carlita was fiddling with the time machine.

Genome hopped in and the time machine was gone in a flash, landing back in the *Mad Scientists' Laboratory*.

Stop them!

It won't click over, but I have an idea. That hospital robot's battery is just what I need. Got it.

CLOSET

Malcolm and Carlita hauled the exhausted Sugar home on the sled. When they reached his window a tap on the shoulder got him to sleepily climb back into his room. Malcolm tucked a copy of *The Healthy Body Treatment Guide* under Sugar's arms.

"How will we know if our plan worked?" asked Carlita.

"That's what the Genome Cam is for," said Malcolm. "Tune in at 0500 hours on your home computer for live video courtesy of our furry detective partner."

Early the next morning, Malcolm and Carlita watched as Sugar awakened.

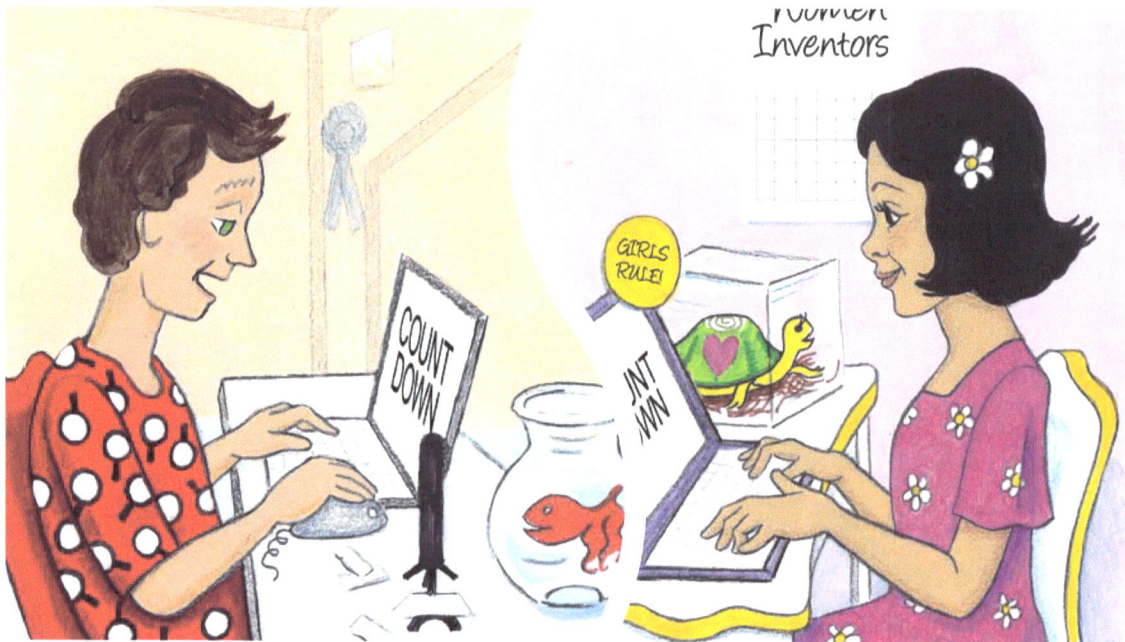

"AHHHHHHH!" screamed Sugar. "NOT MY BIG TOE."

Sugar's mom came running into his room. "What, baby?" she asked. "My goodness, what happened to you?"

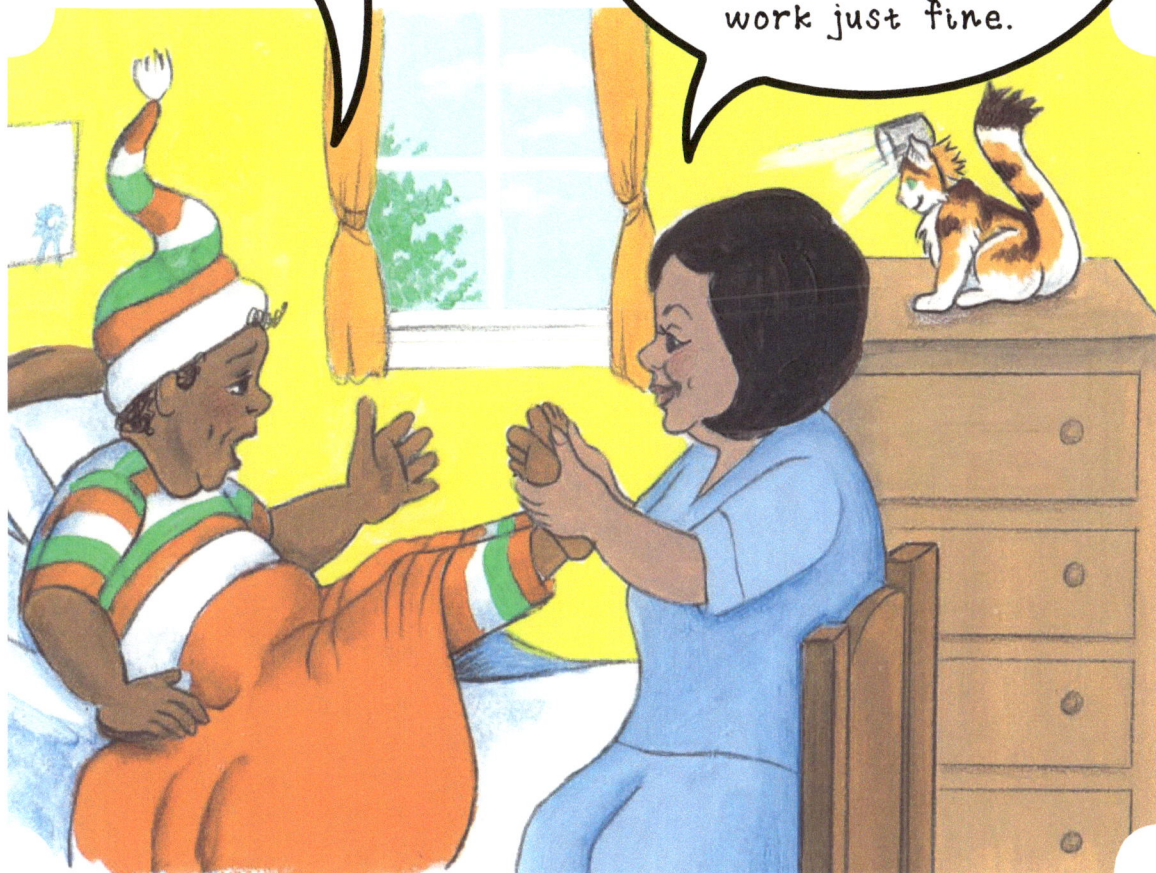

Momma, I don't want to lose my big toe. I don't want to have diabetes. I don't want to be so obese that I can't walk.

Honey, what are you talking about? You have all ten toes. And you're just big-boned like Momma and your brothers. And your legs work just fine.

"I know you love me and that sometimes you say things to make me feel better about myself," said Sugar. "But it's best for me to face the truth. This weight doesn't make me who I am, but it does limit what I can do."

"You're right," said Momma Lee. "Sometimes even we adults don't think about how today can affect tomorrow for our babies."

If I don't change my eating habits and start exercising, this weight will cause me all kinds of problems.

Making some changes would be a good idea. Now come here and give me some sugar.

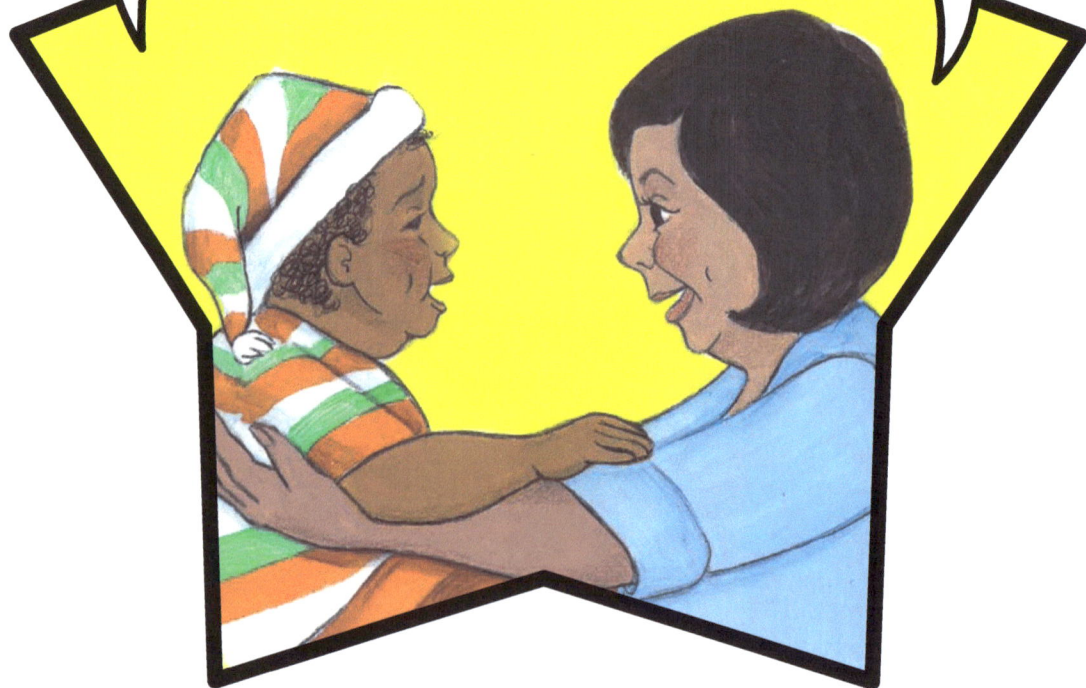

A few weeks later, Malcolm and Carlita spotted Sugar carrying around a very different tray at the Milton Ice Festival. He had changed his business name to *Lee's Treats* and had even changed his portion sizes and products.

"Hey, Sugar!" said Malcolm. "Wow, look at your new selection. Seems like you're getting the hang of eating healthier."

"Boy, am I!" said Sugar. "Thanks to my two favorite detectives, I've learned to make and bake healthier options. Also, with daily family walks and help from your mom, I can avoid medications."

By the way, no one calls me Sugar anymore; they just call me Lee.

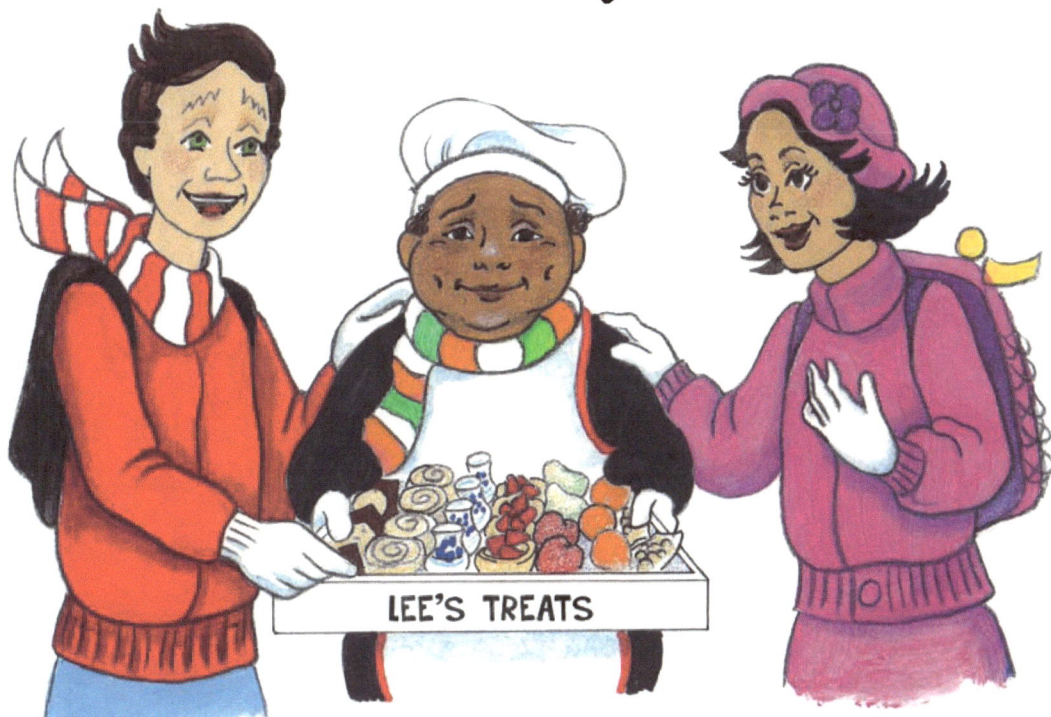

LEE'S TREATS

Malcolm grabbed a bite-size Triple-Chocolate-Threat Brownie from the tray.

I'm sure you're saving that for after a little ice rink exercise and a healthy lunch.

Haha...yeah...of course! Skating, lunch, and then who knows what medical mysteries are in store for us later. Case solved!

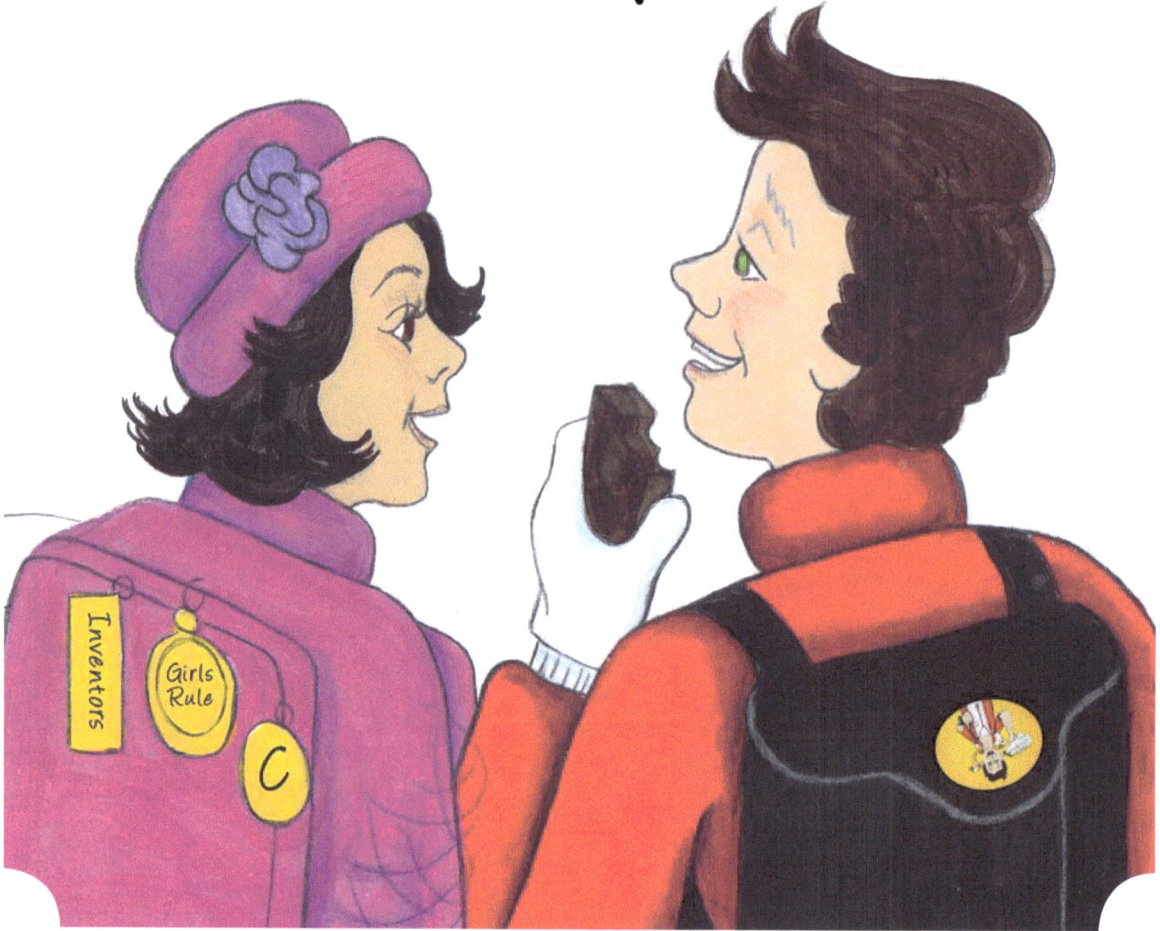

What, what are you staring at? No this isn't kitty fat. Unfortunately I just got a bath so my fur's a bit fuzzy and big today. Besides... beauty shines from the inside out, right? Although, if I ate too many cat treats I might not be able to help Malcolm with all of his wacky adventures, because I wouldn't be able to keep up.

Okay, so maybe being healthy inside is a major part of feeling beautiful on the outside. It would be really hard to be this charming, witty, and handsome if my body wasn't healthy. Looks aren't everything but as Sugar Lee learned; sometimes the way a body looks can indicate body functioning and physical limitations. This can eventually affect how the person feels about themself. You only have one body, so take care of it. And remember, everyone's healthiest body will look different. We are all unique and so are the proportions of our muscles, skin, and fat.

Turn the page to find healthy body resources and meet our author and illustrator. Learn more about childhood obesity and diabetes along with other fun books by logging on to www.bandagesandbooboos.com.

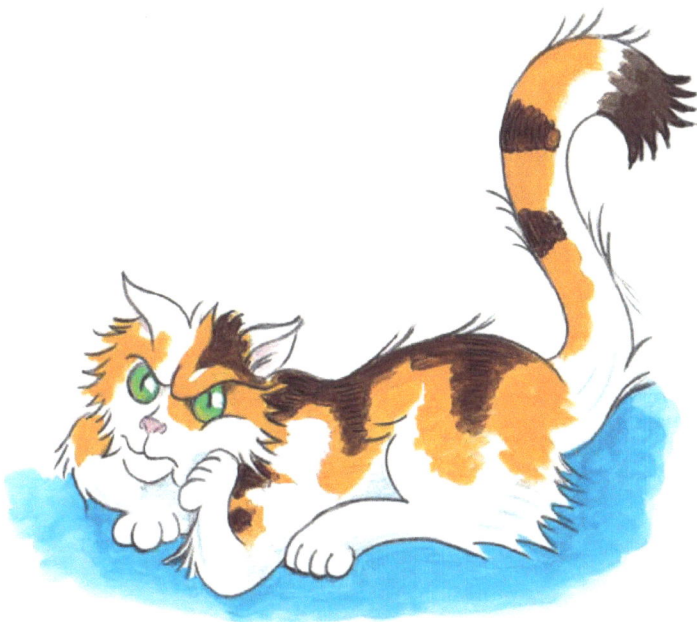

8. GLOSSARY

🐾 **ACINI CELLS:** Cells in the pancreas that make gastric juices to help break down food.

🐾 **ALPHA CELLS:** Pancreatic cells that make glucagon, a hormone that tells the liver to release stored sugar (glycogen) and turn it into ready-to-use sugar (glucose). It tells the rest of the body to burn sources of energy like glucose or fat.

🐾 **BETA CELLS:** Pancreatic cells that make insulin, a hormone that tells the liver to store sugar (glucose) away as glycogen, or for fat storage use.

🐾 **BODY MASS INDEX:** A number that helps figure out if a person is obese. The meaning of this number can be different for children and adults. A special graph is needed to determine healthy body masses for kids.

🐾 **CALORIE:** A unit that measures how much energy food contains. High-fat or high-sugar foods can be very small and have many calories, while even large amounts of low-fat and low-sugar foods can have very few calories. Eating too many calories creates extra fat on the body, but eating too few calories interferes with growth.

🐾 **DIABETES:** A condition where the body doesn't produce insulin (Type 1 Diabetes) or doesn't respond to insulin normally (Type 2 Diabetes). In Type 2 Diabetes, low insulin levels cause a buildup of sugar (glucose) in the blood, which can cause problems in many other organs like the skin, eyes, nerves, heart, kidneys, liver and brain. People with diabetes may feel tired, thirsty and hungry; have itchy, burning, tingly skin and fuzzy vision; and have to use the bathroom a lot.

🐾 **ENDOCRINE:** Glands that produce hormones that are transported in blood or lymph fluid.

🐾 **FAT:** (Adipose tissue). The jiggly blocks that collect underneath skin (subcutaneous fat) or around organs. Fat can serve as an energy reserve, a cushion, or heat insulation.

🐾 **HORMONE:** A chemical messenger made in various body organs that tells other body organs or parts what to do.

🐾 **ISLETS OF LANGERHANS:** The clustered community of alpha, beta, and delta cells in the pancreas.

44

9. THE TREATMENT GUIDE

Obesity and Type 2 Diabetes can result from eating too many calories, not exercising, and gaining weight beyond the norm for a person's age, height and gender. So it makes sense that to reverse these diseases you have to change those actions. It sounds easy enough but bad habits can be hard to change. It takes will-power, physical strength, and love for yourself and those around you, to make changes that will be better for you and your family. Just think about all the things you'll be able to do better, when you are the healthiest you that you can be. But remember, everyone on this earth is made differently and everyone's healthiest body will look different too. Use this guide to start your adventure toward a body that will work for you and let you live your dreams.

FOOD

🐾 **FRUITS AND VEGETABLES (THE MAJOR VITAMIN AND MINERAL GROUP)** Eat first from the earth. The healthiest foods come right out of the dirt with minimal processing (aim for 5 servings a day). Fruits and vegetables should be a large part of your diet. These foods are low in fat, high in fiber, and low in complex carbohydrates. They are a quick snack because many don't require cooking. Set a colorful bowl of fruit out on your kitchen counter to remind you about eating these foods as snacks first, instead of unhealthy foods. If you live in a neighborhood where fresh fruits and vegetables are hard to find at nearby stores, look for local farmers markets.

🐾 **MEAT, POULTRY AND SEAFOOD+ (THE PROTEIN GROUP)** Although fruits and vegetables are awesome foods, they should not be the only items on your plate. Protein is an important nutrient that you get from meats, seafood, beans, and dairy. Cheese and milk are great sources of protein that come packed with valuable calcium and Vitamin D for bones and teeth. Protein is overall an important nutrient in building, maintaining, and replacing tissue in the body.

🐾 **BREADS, GRAINS, AND OTHER STARCHES (THE COMPLEX CARBOHYDRATE GROUP)** Complex carbohydrates do have an important place on the plate. Carbohydrates are typically starchy foods like rice, breads, pasta, cereal, and other items that are usually non-refrigerated. On a perfect plate, these should be present along with a fruit or vegetable and a protein. The best complex carbohydrates are whole grain products, which take longer to break down and help a belly feel full. But beware: if you eat too many carbs they can be stored as fat. Always balance out complex carbohydrates with other food groups.

🐾 **FATS AND SUGARS** Not all fat is evil. A human body needs fat to function normally, especially during childhood. Growing children require higher amounts of fat (30-90 grams daily) than adults do (20-60 grams) to promote brain and nerve growth. The recommended daily fat intake may be easily gained from condiments like butter, syrup, or other items like the occasional bowl of ice cream. But be careful, as sugar can be another concern. Although moderate amounts are naturally found in fruits, most baked goods are made from large amounts of sugar. If you eat too many of them, they could end up as heavy fat cells that burden the body. Again, moderation and balance is the key!

🐾 **PREPARATION OF FOODS** Grilling, steaming and baking are some of the healthiest ways to prepare foods. Frying or sautéing in large amounts of sauce or butter can add extra fat and calories to normally healthy foods. Over-boiling vegetables can remove their natural vitamins and minerals.

🐾 **CALORIES AND PORTION SIZES** Listen to your body and consume the amount of food you need to feel your best. Eat when you are hungry, stop when you feel full, and avoid giving in to unhealthy cravings too often. The right amount of food and calories can vary from person to person. Most kids need between 1600-2500 calories a day, but some kids may need more. If you're concerned, speak with your health care provider about the best calorie intake for your body. Keep your metabolic carburetor going, by eating breakfast, lunch, dinner and snacks in between. Skipping meals can slow metabolism causing you to overeat and make poor food choices. By eating healthy snacks like cheese and fruit between meals, you prevent your belly from getting the grumbles that make you overeat at mealtime. A good rule of thumb is to balance your plate with a protein food the size of your fist (1/4 plate), a starchy carbohydrate (like whole grain rice) the size of a tennis ball (1/4 plate), and a heaping helping of a fresh fruit or vegetable to top it off (1/2 plate).

BEVERAGES

Many flavored beverages contain lots of sugar. High-sugar drinks like soda, punch, and juice can add extra calories with little nutritional value. Limit high-sugar drinks like soda and replace with nutrient packed refreshments like milk or thirst quenchers like water.

PHYSICAL ACTIVITY

Move your body to get your engine burning extra calories you don't need. Find a physical activity you enjoy doing, like karate, gymnastics, hiking, tennis, basketball, or dance. Participating in activities you enjoy will make exercising a lot easier. Look for sports clubs to join at school, a local YMCA, or neighborhood gym. Or just grab your skateboard, roller blades, or bicycle to create your own exercise regimen. Working out with friends may also be a great motivation. Check out your local library for aerobic or dance videos you can do with a group in your own home.

10. GET CONNECTED

1 Start your detective mission off on the right foot by visiting www.bandagesandbooboos.com, where you can clue in to obesity and diabetes facts, figures, contests, and tales. Parents and teachers will also find useful lesson plans that correspond with the Malcolm Finney book series.

2 When you're ready to search for more clues, browse the kid-friendly information at www.kidshealth.org. Under the Staying Healthy tab you can learn more about weight, foods, exercise, and keeping your body healthy. You can also search for more facts about obesity and diabetes.

3 The CDC provides a wealth of useful information about healthy eating, exercise, games and activities on the illustrated pages of BAM (Body and Mind) at www.bam.gov.

4 Www.kidnetic.com contains ideas for fun exercises, active games, and healthy recipes. It also provides easy-to-read articles about things you need to keep healthy.

5 The Let's Move campaign focuses on eliminating obesity by providing and/or promoting educational tools and awareness of healthy food and exercise options on www.letsmove.gov. The goal of this campaign is to provide ideas for increasing physical activity and eating less sugary and unhealthy foods while eating more fruits and vegetables. It also provides information about childhood obesity in our population.

6 The mission outlined on www.foodcorps.org is to "Teach kids about what healthy food is and where it comes from, build and tend school gardens, and bring high-quality local food into public school cafeterias." This is a great resource to help communities put healthy eating habits into action.

Erika Kimble, RN, BSN, MA, MS, CNP

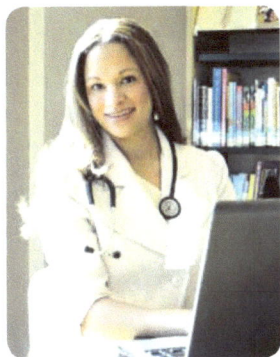

Erika's interest in writing and science began in her elementary years. If she wasn't exploring the woods around her, she was at the library checking out stacks of books. She also penciled away at short stories and poetry.

These childhood pursuits blossomed during her studies at The Ohio State University. After obtaining a Bachelor's in Nursing, Erika spent several years as a Neonatal Intensive Care nurse before deciding to pursue graduate school. Her collegiate years concluded with a Master's in Family Practice as a Nurse Practitioner and a Master's in Journalism and Communications. As a professional in the medical field, she has focused on family health and dermatology. When she's not being a medical detective or writer, Erika enjoys spending time with her two wonderful children and loving husband

Laurel Winters, BFA, MFA

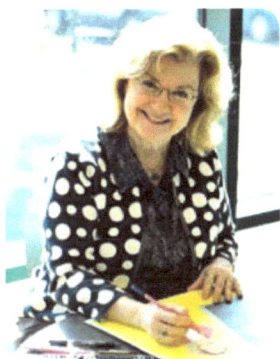

Laurel knew she wanted to be an artist since she was four. Her love of visual expression motivated her to pursue degrees in painting, drawing and printmaking at Virginia Commonwealth University.

Laurel began sharing her passion for art in workshops once her children were in school, eventually teaching art classes from PreK through high school. On the university level, she has taught art education, art history, history of women artists and studio classes. In addition to her paintings, collages and jewelry, she has published magazine and CD covers. The Malcolm Finney series is her first foray into book illustration, completing the cycle she and her husband shared years ago reading bedtime stories to their sons.

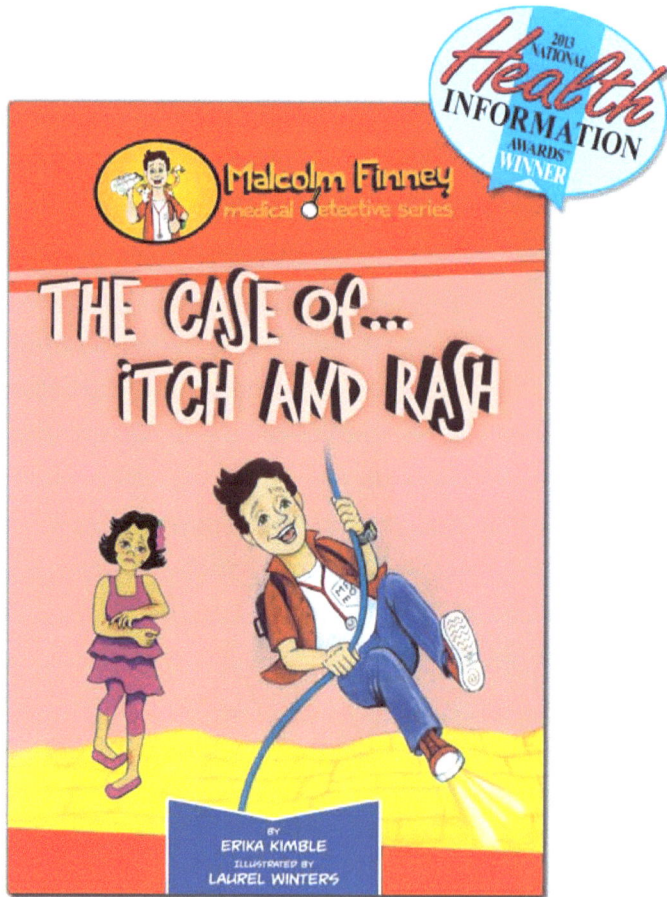

Find our other award winning publication on
www.bandagesandbooboos.com,
www.amazon.com, and **www.barnesandnoble.com**.

www.ingramcontent.com/pod-product-compliance
Lightning Source LLC
Chambersburg PA
CBHW060847270326
41934CB00002B/37